Table of Contents

| *Foreword* |

Into the 21st century, diabetes and heart disease continue to present a challenge. Scientific research and medical advances provide new options to treat these conditions, but the real power to improve your health and that of your family lies in the choices you make every day.

It's up to you: Wise lifestyle choices, such as eating more vegetables and taking a walk every day, do reduce your risk of developing diabetes, heart disease, stroke, and cancer. If you already have diabetes or heart disease (and they go hand in hand), the choices you make will help you manage them both.

The link between diabetes and cardiovascular disease is well established. People with diabetes are two to four times more likely than others to have heart disease or stroke. The good news, however, is that the same things that are good for patients with diabetes are good for those with heart-health issues.

The American Diabetes Association (ADA) and the American Heart Association (AHA) are proud to offer the second edition of our first joint cookbook as we work together to help you live a healthier life. These taste-tested recipes were designed to follow the nutritional guidelines of both the ADA and the AHA. You can choose your meals with confidence, knowing that as you enjoy good food you are also taking care of your heart and your health.

To help you make wise choices, each recipe includes a nutrition analysis of the calories, saturated fat, cholesterol, sodium, and carbohydrates, among other nutrients. Because obesity is the leading risk factor for diabetes and a risk factor for cardiovascular disease (the most serious complication of diabetes), you are wise to eat meals that are lower in calories and unhealthful fats. Use the analyses to tailor your eating plan to your individual needs.

Simple choices add up. These small steps can lead to big changes. Try to eat at least three servings of nonstarchy vegetables a day—a few more is even better. Aim to eat fresh or unsweetened frozen or canned fruit and plenty of whole grains. Stay away from sweetened drinks. Drink more water and zero-calorie drinks. Leave the highly processed white flour, white sugar, and bad fats in the grocery store, and enjoy a journey through the colorful and flavorful world of fresh food prepared lightly. You'll feel so much better when you do.

Here's to your best health!

Robert E. Ratner, MD, FACP, FACE
Chief Scientific and Medical Officer
American Diabetes Association

Rose Marie Robertson, MD, FAHA
Chief Science and Medical Officer
American Heart Association/American Stroke Association

| *Introduction* |

EAT BETTER, FEEL BETTER

Diabetes is a major risk factor for heart disease and stroke. The fact is that adolescents and young adults are developing type 2 diabetes at an alarming rate. The seriousness of this situation as it relates to cardiovascular health prompted the American Heart Association and the American Diabetes Association to join forces in an effort to reverse the trend. Healthful lifestyle choices, especially appropriate diet and daily physical activity, can have a major impact on the prevention and treatment of cardiovascular disease in people with diabetes.

The American Diabetes Association and the American Heart Association want to help you make wise choices about the foods you eat. The American Heart Association has contributed to this book by developing delicious and heart-healthy recipes that meet its dietary recommendations. These recipes also are designed to be consistent with the American Diabetes Association dietary guidelines and will introduce variety into meal plans for people with diabetes.

SIX SIMPLE STEPS TO GOOD HEALTH

By following the guidelines below, you will enjoy the best of nature's bounty and, at the same time, help prevent the cardiovascular consequences of diabetes.

1. **Enjoy a wide variety of nutritious foods in the right amounts from all the food groups:**

   Include plenty of fiber-rich, whole-grain foods.

   Include legumes, nuts, and seeds.

   Include lots of different kinds of vegetables and fruits, especially deeply colored varieties.

   Choose fat-free or low-fat dairy products.

   Select lean meats and skinless poultry.

   Eat fish, preferably fish rich in omega-3 fatty acids (for example, salmon, trout, and tuna), at least twice a week.

2. **Choose a meal plan low in saturated and trans (hydrogenated) fats.** Replace most of these fats with healthful polyunsaturated and mono-unsaturated fats from foods including nuts (such as walnuts, pecans, and almonds) and healthful oils (such as olive, canola, and corn).

3. **Balance your food intake with regular physical activity to maintain a healthful weight.** Aim for at least 150 minutes of moderate-intensity or 75 minutes of vigorous-intensity aerobic physical activity each week. To lose weight, take in fewer calories or burn more by increasing your activity level until you reach your goal.

4. **Limit your daily intake of dietary cholesterol to less than 300 milligrams (mg).**

5. **Keep your intake of sodium to less than 2,300 mg per day.** (If you have coronary heart disease or congestive heart failure, your doctor may recommend lower limits.) The AHA recommends limiting your daily sodium intake to less than 1,500 mg for the greatest effect on blood pressure; high blood pressure is a major risk factor for heart disease.

6. **If you drink alcohol, limit yourself to one drink per day if you are a woman and two drinks per day if you are a man.**

What quantity of foods should be in your healthful meal plan? These serving sizes, based on the dietary exchanges from the ADA, can help you choose appropriately.

1. Grains, Beans, and Starchy Vegetables

One serving =	1 slice of whole-grain bread	1/3 cup cooked whole-grain pasta
	1/2 cup cooked oatmeal, wheat cereal, or polenta	1/2 cup cooked legumes or starchy vegetables, such as pinto beans
	3/4 cup unsweetened flaked cereal	1/2 cup cooked sweet potatoes
	1/3 cup cooked brown rice	

2. Fruits and Vegetables

One serving =	1 small apple, banana, orange, or pear	1/2 cup cooked or chopped vegetables or fruit
	1 cup cubed melon or papaya	1/2 cup 100% fruit juice or vegetable juice
	1 1/4 cups whole strawberries	1 cup raw leafy greens

3. Meat and Meat Substitutes

One serving =	1 ounce fat-free or reduced-fat cheese	1 egg, 2 egg whites, or 1/4 cup egg substitute
	1/2 cup fat-free or low-fat cottage cheese	2 tablespoons low-sodium peanut butter
	4 ounces soy product, such as tofu or soy burger	1 ounce canned very low sodium tuna or salmon or 2 medium sardines (packed in water)
	3 ounces cooked (4 ounces raw) lean meat, poultry, or seafood	

4. Dairy Products

One serving =	1 cup fat-free or low-fat milk	1 cup fat-free or low-fat plain yogurt

5. Fats

One serving =	10 peanuts	1 teaspoon canola or corn oil
	1 tablespoon sesame seeds	2 tablespoons fat-free or low-fat sour cream
	1 teaspoon light tub margarine	

6. Other Carbohydrates

One serving =	1 granola bar	1/3 cup fat-free or low-fat frozen yogurt
	3 gingersnaps	1 small brownie
	5 vanilla wafers	1/8 pumpkin pie

As a general guide to healthy eating, divide the space on your dinner plate into sections. Put a line down the middle of the plate. On one side, divide it again so you have a total of three sections. Fill the largest section (1/2 the plate) with nonstarchy vegetables. In one of the small sections (1/4 of the plate), add starchy foods. In the other small section, include your protein. To round out the meal, add a piece of fruit or 1/2 cup of fruit salad and an 8-ounce glass of fat-free milk. (If you don't drink milk, you can add another small serving of carbohydrates, such as 8 ounces of fat-free yogurt.)

HEART-HEALTHY MEAL PLANNING

You can design your own meal plans using the recipes in this book. To get you started, here's a sample weekly meal plan based on a weekly average of 2,000 calories per day (calories have been rounded to the nearest five).

Sunday

Breakfast (375 cal)	1 serving *Farmers' Market Omelets* (page 158)
	1/2 cup cubed cantaloupe
	1 whole-grain English muffin with 1 teaspoon light tub margarine
	1/2 cup fat-free milk
Snack (310 cal)	6 ounces fat-free plain Greek yogurt with 1/2 cup sliced strawberries 1 ounce sliced almonds, unsalted
	1 medium banana
Lunch (430 cal)	1 serving *Mushroom and Barley Stew* (page 21)
	1 medium Bartlett pear
	1/2 ounce low-fat Swiss cheese
	1/2 ounce chopped walnuts, unsalted
Snack (400 cal)	3 whole-grain crispbreads with 2 tablespoons low-sodium peanut butter
	1 cup fat-free milk
Dinner (500 cal)	1 serving *Roast Turkey with Orange-Spice Rub* (page 83)
	1/2 cup roasted carrots
	2 cups baby spinach with 2 tablespoons homemade vinaigrette
	1 whole-grain dinner roll
	1 serving *Cranberry-Pecan Baked Peaches* (page 171)

Daily Total: 2,015 calories

Monday

Breakfast
(440 cal)
	1 1/4 cups shredded wheat minis with
	    1 cup fat-free milk
	    1/2 cup blueberries
	    1/2 ounce chopped pecans, unsalted

Snack
(200 cal)
	6 ounces fat-free plain Greek yogurt with
	    1/2 cup raspberries
	    1 ounce sliced almonds, unsalted

Lunch (485 cal)	1 serving *Italian Lentil Soup* (page 20)
	1 whole-grain dinner roll with 1 teaspoon light tub margarine
	2 cups baby spinach with 2 tablespoons homemade vinaigrette
	1 medium apple

Snack
(250 cal)
	2 servings *Triple-Duty Ranch Dip with Dill* (page 4) with
	    6 baby carrots
	    6 grape tomatoes
	    4 whole-grain pita wedges, toasted

	1 cup grapes
Dinner (580 cal)	1 serving *Slow-Cooker Mediterranean Pot Roast* (page 91)
	1 serving *Salad Greens with Mixed-Herb Vinaigrette* (page 25)
	1 medium banana

Daily Total: 1,955 calories

Tuesday

Breakfast **(385 cal)**	1 serving *Apple Pie Breakfast Parfaits* (page 160)
	1 whole-grain English muffin with 1 teaspoon light tub margarine
	1/2 cup fat-free milk
Snack **(270 cal)**	6 ounces fat-free plain Greek yogurt with 1 serving *Apricot and Apple Granola* (page 156)
Lunch **(550 cal)**	1 serving *Greek Meatball and Orzo Soup* (page 17)
	2 cups mixed greens with 2 tablespoons homemade vinaigrette
	1/2 6-inch whole-grain pita
	1 medium orange
Snack **(370 cal)**	3 whole-grain crispbreads with 1 1/2 ounces low-fat Swiss cheese
	1 cup grapes
	1 ounce sliced almonds, unsalted
Dinner **(450 cal)**	1 serving *Salmon Tacos* (page 54)
	1/2 cup cooked brown rice
	1 serving *Fanned Avocado Salad* (page 32)
	1 medium peach

Daily Total: 2,025 calories

Wednesday

**Breakfast
(510 cal)**

1 1/4 cups shredded wheat minis with
    1 cup fat-free milk
    1/2 ounce chopped pecans, unsalted

1 medium banana

**Snack
(310 cal)**

6 ounces fat-free plain Greek yogurt with
    1/2 cup mixed berries

2 whole-grain crispbreads with
    1 tablespoon all-fruit spread

**Lunch
(565 cal)**

2 slices whole-grain bread with
    1 serving *Roast Turkey with Orange-Spice Rub* (page 83)
    1 1/2 ounces low-fat Swiss cheese
    1/2 cup dark green lettuce
    2 large slices of tomato
    1 tablespoon light mayonnaise

1 serving *Tomato Basil Bisque* (page 13)

1 medium Bartlett pear

**Snack
(270 cal)**

2 servings *Triple-Duty Ranch Dip with Dill* (page 4) with
    1/2 cup bell pepper strips
    6 baby carrots
    1/2 cup edamame

1/2 ounce dry-roasted, unsalted pistachios

**Dinner
(390 cal)**

1 serving *Stir-Fry Vegetables and Brown Rice* (page 118)

1 serving *Crunchy Asian Snow Pea Salad* (page 28)

1 serving *Fresh Fruit Parfaits* (page 172)

Daily Total: 2,045 calories

Thursday

Breakfast (570 cal)	2 slices whole-grain toast with 2 teaspoons light tub margarine
	6 ounces fat-free plain Greek yogurt with 1/2 cup mixed berries 2 tablespoons chopped walnuts, unsalted
	1 cup fat-free milk
Snack (170 cal)	1 1/2 ounces low-fat Swiss cheese
	1 medium Bartlett pear
Lunch (350 cal)	1 serving *Chicken Antipasto Salad* (page 39) on 1 cup mixed greens
	1 medium orange
Snack (260 cal)	1 serving *Apricot and Apple Granola* (page 156) with 3 cups air-popped popcorn
Dinner (600 cal)	1 serving *Vegetable Chili with Mixed Beans* (page 124) over 3/4 cup cooked barley
	1 serving *Caribbean Fruit Salad Platter* (page 34)
	1 whole-grain dinner roll

Daily Total: 1,950 calories

Friday

Breakfast (535 cal)	1 serving *Apricot and Apple Granola* (page 156) with 1 cup fat-free milk
	1 whole-grain English muffin with 1 teaspoon light tub margarine
	1 cup fresh orange juice
Snack (390 cal)	1 medium banana with 2 tablespoons low-sodium peanut butter
	1 cup fat-free milk
Lunch (500 cal)	1 serving *Cranberry-Pecan Turkey Salad* (page 40)
	2 cups baby spinach with 2 tablespoons homemade vinaigrette
	1/2 6-inch whole-grain pita
Snack (90 cal)	3 cups air-popped popcorn
Dinner (490 cal)	1 serving *Grilled Trout Amandine with Ginger and Orange* (page 58)
	1 serving *Toasted-Almond Rice and Peas* (page 133)
	8 medium grilled asparagus spears
	2 slices grilled pineapple

Daily Total: 2,005 calories

Saturday

Breakfast (360 cal)	1 serving *Southwestern Breakfast Tortilla Wraps* (page 159)
	1 cup grapes
	1 cup fat-free milk
Snack (470 cal)	3 whole-grain crispbreads with 1 1/2 ounces low-fat Swiss cheese
	1 medium apple with 2 tablespoons low-sodium peanut butter
Lunch (545 cal)	1 serving *Broccoli Cheese Soup* (page 12)
	2 slices whole-grain bread with 3 ounces very low sodium albacore tuna, packed in water 1 tablespoon light mayonnaise 1/2 cup dark green lettuce 2 large slices of tomato
	1 medium orange
Snack (280 cal)	2 servings *Spinach and Artichoke Dip* (page 3) with 8 whole-grain pita wedges, toasted
	2 cups air-popped popcorn with 1/2 ounce dry-roasted, unsalted pistachios
Dinner (360 cal)	1 serving *Roasted-Veggie Pizza on a Phyllo Crust* (page 112)
	1 serving *Mixed Green Salad with Peppery Citrus Dressing* (page 24)
	1 serving *Minted Fruit Ice* (page 176) with 1/2 small cantaloupe

Daily Total: 2,015 calories

HOW TO USE THE RECIPE ANALYSES

To help you with meal planning, we have carefully analyzed each recipe in this cookbook to provide useful nutrition information. If your healthcare professional has told you to restrict the amount of sodium or saturated fat in your meal plan, read the analyses and choose your recipes carefully.

Each analysis is based on one serving of the dish, unless otherwise indicated, and includes all the ingredients listed. Optional ingredients and garnishes, however, are not analyzed unless otherwise noted; neither are foods suggested as accompaniments.

We've made every effort to provide accurate nutrition information. Because of the many variables involved in analyzing foods, however, these values should be considered approximate.

When a recipe lists ingredient options, such as 1/2 cup fat-free or low-fat cheddar cheese, we analyzed the first one.

Values except for fats are rounded to the nearest whole number. Fat values are rounded to the nearest gram. The values for saturated, monounsaturated, and polyunsaturated fats are rounded to the nearest 0.1 gram. These values may not add up to the total fat in the recipe, because total fat also includes other fatty substances and glycerol.

We used canola, corn, and olive oil in our recipes, but you can use any other oil with no more than 2 grams of saturated fat per tablespoon—safflower, sunflower, sesame, soybean, walnut, or almond.

We used healthful oils and light tub margarine as our preferred fats and used stick margarine sparingly. When selecting a stick margarine, choose one that lists liquid vegetable oil as the first ingredient. It should contain no more than 2 grams of saturated fat per tablespoon and should be trans fat free. We used corn oil stick margarine for the analysis.

Meats are analyzed as cooked and lean, with all visible fat discarded. Values for ground beef are based on meat that is 95 percent fat free.

If meat, poultry, or seafood is marinated and the marinade is discarded, we calculated only the amount of marinade absorbed. We calculated the total amount of the marinade used in marinated vegetables. We did the same for liquids used for basting or dipping.

The specific ingredients listed in each recipe were analyzed. For instance, we used both fat-free and low-fat cheddar cheese in this collection of recipes, depending on the taste and texture desired. In each case, the type listed was used for the nutrition analysis. If you prefer a different variety, use it. Of course, the fat values will change with such substitutions. Other nutrient values, such as sodium, may change as well. On the other hand, if you want to substitute reconstituted lemon juice for fresh, or white onions for yellow, the substitutions won't change the ingredient analyses enough to matter.

We use the abbreviations "g" for gram and "mg" for milligram.

| *Appetizers and Snacks* |

LAYERED FIESTA BEAN DIP

Serves 20 / Serving Size: 2 tablespoons

Fat-free refried beans form the base of this healthy update on a party classic. They're topped with tangy sour cream and a fresh pico de gallo and then sprinkled with cheddar. Baked, unsalted tortilla chips or strips of red and yellow bell peppers are deliciously appropriate dippers.

1/2 (15.5-ounce) can fat-free refried beans or 1/2 (15.5-ounce) can no-salt-added pinto beans, rinsed, drained, and mashed with a potato masher

1/4 cup salsa (lowest sodium available)

1/8 teaspoon salt

1/2 cup fat-free sour cream

1 medium Italian plum (Roma) tomato, diced

1/4 small onion, finely chopped

1/8 cup loosely packed fresh cilantro, coarsely chopped

1 1/2 teaspoons fresh lime juice

1/2 small fresh jalapeño, seeds and ribs discarded, coarsely chopped (optional)

1/4 cup shredded fat-free cheddar cheese

Exchanges / Choices
1 Vegetable

Calories	20	**Sodium**	115 mg
Calories from Fat	0	**Potassium**	85 mg
Total Fat	**0 g**	**Total Carbohydrate**	**4 g**
Saturated Fat	0 g	Dietary Fiber	1 g
Trans Fat	0 g	Sugars	1 g
Polyunsaturated Fat	0 g	**Protein**	**1 g**
Monounsaturated Fat	0 g	**Phosphorus**	**40 mg**
Cholesterol	**0 mg**		

1. In a medium bowl, stir together the beans, salsa, and salt. Spread in an 8-inch square glass baking dish or serving dish.

2. Spread the sour cream over the bean mixture.

3. In a small bowl, stir together the remaining ingredients except the cheddar. Spread over the sour cream. Sprinkle with the cheddar.

SPINACH AND ARTICHOKE DIP

Serves 26 / Serving Size: 2 tablespoons

This creamy dip gets a surprising bit of bite from a small amount of horseradish. And it's loaded with tasty morsels of artichoke hearts, spinach, roasted red bell peppers, and green onions, making it a breeze to sneak some extra vegetables into your diet. Serve it with whole-grain pita chips or endive leaves for dipping, or spread it on triangles of whole-grain toast.

12 ounces frozen artichoke hearts, thawed and chopped

1 1/2 cups fat-free plain Greek yogurt

10 ounces frozen chopped spinach, thawed and squeezed dry

1/2 cup shredded or grated Parmesan cheese

1/2 cup chopped roasted red bell peppers, drained if bottled

2 medium green onions, thinly sliced

1 tablespoon dried minced onion or 1 teaspoon onion powder

1 teaspoon bottled white horseradish, drained (optional)

1/2 teaspoon garlic powder

1/8 teaspoon salt

1/8 teaspoon red hot-pepper sauce

Exchanges / Choices			
1 Vegetable			

Calories	30	Sodium	100 mg
Calories from Fat	5	Potassium	105 mg
Total Fat	**0.5 g**	**Total Carbohydrate**	**3 g**
Saturated Fat	0.5 g	Dietary Fiber	1 g
Trans Fat	0 g	Sugars	1 g
Polyunsaturated Fat	0 g	**Protein**	**3 g**
Monounsaturated Fat	0 g	**Phosphorus**	**45 mg**
Cholesterol	**0 mg**		

1. In a medium bowl, stir together all the ingredients. Cover and refrigerate for at least 30 minutes, or until the minced onion has softened.

TRIPLE-DUTY RANCH DIP WITH DILL

Serves 16 / Serving Size: 2 tablespoons

Dunk crisp carrot and celery sticks, broccoli florets, or even cucumber rounds into this cool dip. It also serves beautifully as a salad dressing or as a sauce for broiled or poached salmon, and it pairs perfectly with our Tex-Mex Chicken Fingers (page 71).

1 cup low-fat buttermilk

1 cup fat-free sour cream

1 tablespoon chopped fresh dillweed
or 1 teaspoon dried dillweed, crumbled

1 tablespoon chopped green onions (green part only)

1 tablespoon chopped fresh parsley or
1 teaspoon dried parsley, crumbled

1 teaspoon onion powder

1/2 teaspoon garlic powder

1/2 teaspoon dry mustard

1/2 teaspoon pepper (coarsely ground preferred)

1/8 teaspoon salt

1. In a medium bowl, whisk together all the ingredients. Cover and refrigerate for at least 30 minutes before serving.

Exchanges / Choices
1 Vegetable

Calories	20	**Sodium**	50 mg
Calories from Fat	0	**Potassium**	60 mg
Total Fat	0 g	**Total Carbohydrate**	4 g
Saturated Fat	0 g	Dietary Fiber	<1 g
Trans Fat	0 g	Sugars	1 g
Polyunsaturated Fat	1 g	**Protein**	1 g
Monounsaturated Fat	0 g	**Phosphorus**	30 mg
Cholesterol	0 mg		

DIJON DIP WITH TARRAGON

Serves 6 / Serving Size: 2 tablespoons

Pungent Dijon mustard and aromatic tarragon make a sophisticated pairing in this smooth dip. It's a tangy accompaniment to crudités, but be sure and try it as a tasty sandwich spread, too.

1/2 cup fat-free plain Greek yogurt

2 tablespoons light mayonnaise

1 tablespoon Dijon mustard (lowest sodium available)

2 teaspoons olive oil (extra virgin preferred)

1 1/4 teaspoons dried tarragon, crumbled

1/2 medium garlic clove, minced

1/8 teaspoon salt

1. In a small bowl, whisk together all the ingredients until smooth.

Exchanges / Choices			
1 Fat			

Calories	40	**Sodium**	140 mg
Calories from Fat	30	**Potassium**	40 mg
Total Fat	**3 g**	**Total Carbohydrate**	**1 g**
Saturated Fat	0.5 g	Dietary Fiber	<1 g
Trans Fat	0 g	Sugars	1 g
Polyunsaturated Fat	1 g	**Protein**	**2 g**
Monounsaturated Fat	1.5 g	**Phosphorus**	30 mg
Cholesterol	**0 mg**		

PEACH AND PINEAPPLE SPREAD

Serves 20 / Serving Size: 2 tablespoons

For a double dose of ginger, try this fruit spread on low-fat gingersnaps. Its slight spiciness provides a perfect foil for the sweetness of peaches and pineapple, while light tub cream cheese gives it a velvety texture.

1 (14.5-ounce) can sliced peaches canned in water, drained

1 cup drained pineapple chunks canned in their own juice

8 ounces light tub cream cheese, softened

1 tablespoon honey

1/4 teaspoon ground ginger

1/8 teaspoon ground nutmeg

1. In a food processor or blender, process all the ingredients to the desired texture (either smooth or slightly chunky). Transfer to a serving bowl.

Cook's Tip: Try this summery spread on toasted whole-grain bread for breakfast or on low-fat graham crackers for a quick snack that will satisfy your sweet tooth in a heart-healthy way.

Exchanges / Choices

1/2 Fruit

Calories	40	Sodium	55 mg
Calories from Fat	15	Potassium	30 mg
Total Fat	1.5 g	Total Carbohydrate	6 g
Saturated Fat	1 g	Dietary Fiber	<1 g
Trans Fat	0 g	Sugars	5 g
Polyunsaturated Fat	0 g	Protein	1 g
Monounsaturated Fat	0.5 g	Phosphorus	20 mg
Cholesterol	5 mg		

FRESH TOMATILLO-POBLANO SALSA WITH TORTILLA WEDGES

Serves 6 / Serving Size: 2 tablespoons salsa and 6 tortilla wedges

Sometimes known as Mexican green tomatoes, tomatillos (tohm-ah-TEE-ohs) give this salsa an unexpected tang and hue, while the poblano pepper adds a mild heat. Crisp baked corn tortilla wedges are the perfect scoops.

6 (6-inch) corn tortillas, each cut into 6 wedges

Cooking spray

Salsa

2 medium tomatillos (about 6 ounces total), papery husks discarded

1/2 medium poblano pepper

1/4 cup chopped fresh cilantro

1/8 teaspoon salt

1 tablespoon olive oil (extra virgin preferred)

1. Preheat the oven to 425°F.

2. Arrange the tortilla wedges in a single layer on a large baking sheet. Lightly spray them with cooking spray. Bake for 8–12 minutes, or until lightly browned and crisp, turning once halfway through (watch carefully to make sure they don't burn). Transfer the baking sheet to a cooling rack and let the wedges cool completely, about 5 minutes.

3. In a food processor or blender, process the salsa ingredients except the oil for 10–15 seconds, or until the desired consistency. Pour into a small bowl. Stir in the oil. Serve with the tortilla wedges.

Cook's Tip: For a milder salsa, discard some or all of the seeds and ribs of the poblano before processing it. Refrigerate any remaining salsa in an airtight container for up to two days. Store the tortilla wedges in an airtight container at room temperature for up to one week.

Exchanges / Choices
1 Starch, 1/2 Fat

Calories	90	Sodium	45 mg
Calories from Fat	30	Potassium	100 mg
Total Fat	**3.5 g**	**Total Carbohydrate**	**13 g**
Saturated Fat	0.5 g	Dietary Fiber	2 g
Trans Fat	0 g	Sugars	1 g
Polyunsaturated Fat	1 g	**Protein**	**2 g**
Monounsaturated Fat	2 g	**Phosphorus**	**85 mg**
Cholesterol	**0 mg**		

STUFFED MUSHROOMS WITH HAM AND VEGETABLES

Serves 8 / Serving Size: 4 mushrooms

Every bite of these mushroom morsels boasts a burst of flavor from juicy ham, shredded carrot, and minced green onion. The crunchy walnuts add texture and the chili sauce lends a hint of spice.

32 small button mushrooms (about 1 pound), stems removed and finely chopped

Cooking spray

1 medium carrot, shredded

2 ounces lower-sodium, low-fat ham, all visible fat discarded, diced

1 slice whole-grain bread (lowest sodium available), toasted and diced

1/4 cup shredded or grated Parmesan cheese

1 large egg

2 tablespoons diced walnuts, dry-roasted

1 medium green onion, finely minced

1 tablespoon chili sauce (lowest sodium available)

Exchanges / Choices			
1/2 Carbohydrate, 1 Lean Meat			
Calories	80	Sodium	130 mg
Calories from Fat	30	Potassium	490 mg
Total Fat	**3.5 g**	**Total Carbohydrate**	**6 g**
Saturated Fat	1 g	Dietary Fiber	2 g
Trans Fat	0 g	Sugars	3 g
Polyunsaturated Fat	0 g	**Protein**	**8 g**
Monounsaturated Fat	1.5 g	Phosphorus	170 mg
Cholesterol	**30 mg**		

1. Preheat the oven to 350°F. Line a large baking sheet with aluminum foil.

2. Put the mushrooms with the cap side up on the baking sheet. Lightly spray the caps with cooking spray. Turn the mushrooms over.

3. In a medium bowl, stir together the chopped mushroom stems and the remaining ingredients. Spoon about 2 teaspoons of the mixture into the cavity of each mushroom.

4. Bake for 25–30 minutes, or until the mushrooms are tender and the filling is heated through.

SPINACH-PARMESAN QUICHE BITES

Serves 8 / Serving Size: 2 quiche bites

Serve these mini quiches as a savory snack or an elegant appetizer. Roasted red bell peppers brighten up the classic combination of spinach and Parmesan. These quiches are so flavorful, you'll never miss the crust! *(See photo insert.)*

Cooking spray

10 ounces frozen chopped spinach, thawed and squeezed dry

1/4 cup chopped roasted red bell peppers, drained if bottled

2 medium green onions, thinly sliced

1 tablespoon plus 1 teaspoon shredded or grated Parmesan cheese

1 cup egg substitute

1/2 cup fat-free milk

1 teaspoon dry mustard

1/8 teaspoon salt

1/8 teaspoon pepper

1. Preheat the oven to 350°F. Lightly spray 16 cups of two 12-cup mini muffin pans or 16 cups of a 24-cup mini muffin pan with cooking spray.

2. In a medium bowl, using a fork, separate the spinach into small pieces. Stir in the roasted peppers and green onions. Spoon the spinach mixture into the sprayed muffin cups. Sprinkle the Parmesan over the spinach mixture.

3. In a separate medium bowl, whisk together the remaining ingredients. Pour into the filled muffin cups. Fill the empty muffin cups with water to keep the pan from warping.

4. Bake for 18–20 minutes, or until a wooden toothpick inserted in the center comes out clean. Transfer the pans to a cooling rack. Let cool for 10 minutes. Using a thin spatula or flat knife, loosen the sides of the quiche bites. Serve warm.

5. Refrigerate leftovers in an airtight container for up to five days. To reheat, put 4–6 quiche bites on a microwaveable plate. Microwave on 100% power (high) for 45 seconds–1 minute, or until heated through.

Exchanges / Choices
1 Vegetable, 1 Lean Meat

Calories	50	**Sodium**	190 mg
Calories from Fat	15	**Potassium**	270 mg
Total Fat	1.5 g	**Total Carbohydrate**	3 g
Saturated Fat	0.5 g	Dietary Fiber	1 g
Trans Fat	0 g	Sugars	1 g
Polyunsaturated Fat	1 g	**Protein**	6 g
Monounsaturated Fat	0.5 g	**Phosphorus**	80 mg
Cholesterol	0 mg		

BONELESS BARBECUE "WINGS"

Serves 14 / Serving Size: 2 pieces chicken and scant 1 1/2 teaspoons sauce

Boneless chicken breast meat with a crunchy baked coating stands in for traditional chicken wings in this easy-to-prepare recipe. An enhanced barbecue sauce gives it a spicy-sweet appeal. *(See photo insert.)*

Cooking spray

2 tablespoons whole-wheat flour or all-purpose flour

1/4 teaspoon salt-free seasoned pepper blend

1/4 cup low-fat buttermilk

1 teaspoon red hot-pepper sauce

1 cup crushed corn flake cereal (about 2 1/2 cups flakes)

1 pound boneless, skinless chicken breasts, all visible fat discarded, cut into 28 strips

1/4 cup barbecue sauce (lowest sodium available)

1 tablespoon cider vinegar

1 tablespoon honey

1. Preheat the oven to 350°F. Lightly spray a baking sheet with cooking spray.

2. In a medium shallow dish, stir together the flour and seasoned pepper blend. In a second shallow dish, whisk together the buttermilk and hot-pepper sauce. Put the corn flake crumbs in a third shallow dish. Set the dishes and baking sheet in a row, assembly-line fashion. Working in batches, dip the chicken in the flour mixture, then in the buttermilk mixture, and finally in the corn flake mixture, turning to coat at each step and gently shaking off any excess. Using your fingertips, gently press the coating mixture so it adheres to the chicken.

3. Arrange the chicken in a single layer on the baking sheet. Lightly spray the top of the chicken with cooking spray.

4. Bake for 25 minutes, or until the chicken is no longer pink in the center and the coating is crisp.

5. Meanwhile, in a medium bowl, whisk together the barbecue sauce, vinegar, and honey.

6. Add the chicken to the sauce, stirring gently to coat, or serve the sauce on the side.

Exchanges / Choices
1/2 Carbohydrate, 1 Lean Meat

Calories	75	Sodium	90 mg
Calories from Fat	10	Potassium	150 mg
Total Fat	**1 g**	**Total Carbohydrate**	**8 g**
Saturated Fat	0 g	Dietary Fiber	<1 g
Trans Fat	0 g	Sugars	3 g
Polyunsaturated Fat	0 g	**Protein**	**8 g**
Monounsaturated Fat	0.5 g	Phosphorus	80 mg
Cholesterol	**20 mg**		

| *Soups* |

Broccoli Cheese Soup	12
Tomato Basil Bisque	13
Creamy Caramelized Onion Soup	14
Asian Chicken and Vegetable Stew	15
Split Pea and Lima Bean Soup with Chicken	16
Greek Meatball and Orzo Soup	17
Home-Style Vegetable Beef Soup	18
Pork, Barley, and Vegetable Stew	19
Italian Lentil Soup	20
Mushroom and Barley Stew	21
Vegetable Stew with Fresh Rosemary	22

BROCCOLI CHEESE SOUP

Serves 8 / Serving Size: 3/4 cup

This creamy soup is full of fresh, wholesome broccoli—and lots of flavor, thanks to a combo of cheddar and Parmesan cheeses. For a light lunch, serve the soup with a spinach salad and a crusty whole-grain roll.

1 teaspoon canola or corn oil

1 small onion, finely chopped

2 medium garlic cloves, minced

1 pound broccoli florets, chopped (about 4 cups)

2 cups fat-free, low-sodium chicken or vegetable broth

1/2 teaspoon dry mustard

1/4 teaspoon pepper

1/8 teaspoon red hot-pepper sauce (optional)

1/16 teaspoon salt

2 cups fat-free milk

1/3 cup all-purpose flour

1/2 cup fat-free half-and-half

2 ounces low-fat cheddar cheese, sliced or shredded

2 tablespoons shredded or grated Parmesan cheese

1. In a large saucepan, heat the oil over medium heat, swirling to coat the bottom. Cook the onion and garlic for 3–4 minutes, or until the onion is almost soft, stirring frequently.

2. Stir in the broccoli, broth, mustard, pepper, hot-pepper sauce, and salt. Increase the heat to medium high and bring to a simmer. Reduce the heat and simmer for 5 minutes, or until the broccoli is tender, stirring occasionally.

3. In a medium bowl, whisk together the milk and flour. Stir into the soup. Simmer for 2–3 minutes, or until the mixture has thickened, stirring occasionally.

4. Stir in the half-and-half, cheddar, and Parmesan. Cook over medium-low heat for 1–2 minutes, or until the cheeses have melted, stirring occasionally.

Exchanges / Choices
2 Vegetable, 1/2 Fat-Free Milk

Calories	110	**Sodium**	160 mg
Calories from Fat	25	**Potassium**	390 mg
Total Fat	**2.5 g**	**Total Carbohydrate**	**16 g**
Saturated Fat	1 g	Dietary Fiber	2 g
Trans Fat	0 g	Sugars	7 g
Polyunsaturated Fat	0.5 g	**Protein**	**8 g**
Monounsaturated Fat	1 g	**Phosphorus**	**195 mg**
Cholesterol	**5 mg**		

TOMATO BASIL BISQUE

Serves 8 / Serving Size: 3/4 cup

Fresh basil flavors every spoonful of this smooth soup that can be served warm or chilled. The leeks offer a more subtle taste than onions, but either will work. Try this bisque with a slice of Rosemary Quick Bread (page 154) for a light snack or with a low-fat grilled cheese sandwich on whole-grain bread for lunch.

1 cup fat-free, low-sodium chicken or vegetable broth, divided use

2 medium leeks (white part only), thinly sliced, or 1/2 cup sliced onion

1 small rib of celery, diced

2 medium garlic cloves, minced

1/4 teaspoon salt

1/4 teaspoon pepper

2 pounds tomatoes

1/4 cup loosely packed fresh basil

1/2 cup fat-free half-and-half

1. In a large saucepan, stir together 1/2 cup broth, the leeks, celery, garlic, salt, and pepper. Bring to a simmer over medium-high heat. Reduce the heat and simmer, covered, for 5 minutes, or until the vegetables are tender. Remove from the heat. Let cool for 5 minutes.

2. In a food processor or blender (vent the blender lid), process the leek mixture for about 1 minute, or until smooth. Return the leek mixture to the pan. Keep warm over low heat (uncovered).

3. Fill a small saucepan half-full with cold water. Bring to a boil over high heat. Reduce the heat to medium high. Cut a small X on the bottom of each tomato so the skin will loosen more easily. Put 2 tomatoes in the saucepan. Simmer for 10 seconds, or until the peel starts to loosen from the flesh. Transfer to a cutting board. Repeat with the remaining tomatoes. Let the tomatoes cool for a few minutes. Remove the peel if desired. Cut the tomatoes into four wedges each.

4. In a food processor or blender, process the tomatoes and the remaining 1/2 cup broth in batches until smooth, about 1 minute per batch. Before processing the last batch, add the basil.

5. Stir the tomato mixture into the leek mixture. Increase the heat to medium high and bring to a simmer. Reduce the heat and simmer, partially covered, for 8–10 minutes, stirring occasionally.

6. Stir in the half-and-half. Cook over low heat for 1–2 minutes, or until the soup is heated through, stirring occasionally. Serve warm or refrigerate in an airtight container until chilled.

Exchanges / Choices
2 Vegetable

Calories	50	**Sodium**	90 mg
Calories from Fat	10	**Potassium**	415 mg
Total Fat	1 g	**Total Carbohydrate**	10 g
Saturated Fat	0 g	Dietary Fiber	2 g
Trans Fat	0 g	Sugars	5 g
Polyunsaturated Fat	0 g	**Protein**	3 g
Monounsaturated Fat	0 g	**Phosphorus**	75 mg
Cholesterol	0 mg		

CREAMY CARAMELIZED ONION SOUP

Serves 8 / Serving Size: 3/4 cup

Classic onion soup gets an extra touch of richness in this lush version. It makes an excellent appetizer or a satisfying lunch paired with a sandwich made with leftover Roast Turkey with Orange-Spice Rub (page 83).

1 teaspoon olive oil

2 large onions, thinly sliced

1/4 teaspoon salt

1/4 teaspoon sugar

2 medium garlic cloves, minced

4 cups fat-free, low-sodium chicken broth

1/4 teaspoon pepper

1 cup fat-free half-and-half

1/3 cup all-purpose flour

Exchanges / Choices

1/2 Carbohydrate, 2 Vegetable

Calories	90	Sodium	125 mg
Calories from Fat	20	Potassium	275 mg
Total Fat	**2 g**	**Total Carbohydrate**	**15 g**
Saturated Fat	0.5 g	Dietary Fiber	1 g
Trans Fat	0 g	Sugars	6 g
Polyunsaturated Fat	0 g	**Protein**	**4 g**
Monounsaturated Fat	1 g	Phosphorus	110 mg
Cholesterol	**<5 mg**		

1. In a large saucepan, heat the oil over medium-high heat, swirling to coat the bottom. Cook the onions for 2 minutes, stirring occasionally.

2. Stir in the salt and sugar. Cook for 7–10 minutes, or until the onions are a deep, golden brown, stirring occasionally.

3. Stir in the garlic. Cook for 30 seconds, or until tender, stirring occasionally. Stir in the broth and pepper. Bring to a simmer. Reduce the heat and simmer for 10 minutes, or until the onions are tender.

4. In a medium bowl, whisk together the half-and-half and flour. Stir the mixture into the soup. Increase the heat to medium high. Cook for 3–4 minutes, or until the soup has thickened, stirring occasionally.

ASIAN CHICKEN AND VEGETABLE STEW

Serves 4 / Serving Size: 1 1/4 cups

Tender cubes of chicken, crisp vegetables, and an Asian-inspired broth make for an aromatic entrée. Crunchy Asian Snow Pea Salad (page 28) is a delicious partner.

1 teaspoon toasted sesame oil

1 pound boneless, skinless chicken breasts, all visible fat discarded, cut into 3/4-inch cubes

1 3/4 cups fat-free, low-sodium chicken broth

1 8-ounce can bamboo shoots, rinsed and drained

4 ounces snow peas, trimmed

1/3 cup water and 1 tablespoon water, divided use

4 medium green onions, sliced

3 tablespoons plain rice vinegar

1 1/2 tablespoons soy sauce (lowest sodium available)

1 tablespoon coarsely chopped peeled gingerroot

1 teaspoon light brown sugar

1/4 teaspoon crushed red pepper flakes

1/4 teaspoon pepper

1 tablespoon cornstarch

1. In a large saucepan, heat the oil over medium-high heat, swirling to coat the bottom. Cook the chicken for 6–8 minutes, or until no longer pink in the center, stirring frequently.

2. Stir in the broth, bamboo shoots, snow peas, 1/3 cup water, the green onions, vinegar, soy sauce, gingerroot, brown sugar, red pepper flakes, and pepper. Increase the heat to high and bring to a boil, stirring occasionally. Reduce the heat and simmer for 6–8 minutes, stirring occasionally.

3. Put the cornstarch in a small bowl. Add the remaining 1 tablespoon water, stirring to dissolve. Stir into the soup. Increase the heat to medium high and bring to a boil. Boil for 1–2 minutes, or until thickened, stirring occasionally.

Cook's Tip on Toasted Sesame Oil: Toasted sesame oil provides the authentic Asian flavor in this recipe. Also known as Asian sesame oil, it is darker and has a stronger flavor than regular sesame oil, which is virtually flavorless.

Exchanges / Choices
1/2 Carbohydrate, 1 Vegetable, 3 Lean Meat

Calories	210	Sodium	395 mg
Calories from Fat	45	Potassium	940 mg
Total Fat	**5 g**	**Total Carbohydrate**	**11 g**
Saturated Fat	1 g	Dietary Fiber	3 g
Trans Fat	0 g	Sugars	5 g
Polyunsaturated Fat	1 g	**Protein**	**29 g**
Monounsaturated Fat	1.5 g	**Phosphorus**	**335 mg**
Cholesterol	**70 mg**		

SPLIT PEA AND LIMA BEAN SOUP WITH CHICKEN

Serves 6 / Serving Size: 1 1/2 cups

This hearty soup features two legumes along with robust chunks of chicken and plump baby carrots. Serve it with a crisp salad of mixed lettuces and juicy tomatoes or Tomato Salad with Creamy Horseradish Dressing (page 26).

4 cups water

2 cups fat-free, low-sodium chicken broth

1 cup dried split peas, sorted for stones and shriveled peas, rinsed, and drained

1 pound boneless, skinless chicken breasts, all visible fat discarded, cut into 3/4-inch cubes

2 cups baby carrots

1 (15.5-ounce) can no-salt-added lima beans, rinsed and drained, or 1 3/4 cups frozen lima beans

2 medium ribs of celery, cut into 1/2-inch slices

2 teaspoons onion powder

1 teaspoon dried thyme, crumbled

1 teaspoon dried marjoram, crumbled

1/4 teaspoon salt

1/4 teaspoon pepper

Exchanges / Choices

2 Starch, 1 Vegetable, 3 Lean Meat

Calories	310	**Sodium**	260 mg
Calories from Fat	30	**Potassium**	1090 mg
Total Fat	3.5 g	**Total Carbohydrate**	40 g
Saturated Fat	1 g	Dietary Fiber	5 g
Trans Fat	0 g	Sugars	3 g
Polyunsaturated Fat	1 g	**Protein**	30 g
Monounsaturated Fat	1 g	**Phosphorus**	355 mg
Cholesterol	50 mg		

1. In a stockpot or Dutch oven, bring the water, broth, and peas to a boil over high heat, stirring occasionally. Reduce the heat and simmer, covered, for 45 minutes, or until the peas are almost tender (no stirring needed).

2. Stir in the remaining ingredients. Simmer, covered, for 30–40 minutes, or until the peas and carrots are tender and the chicken is no longer pink in the center, stirring occasionally.

GREEK MEATBALL AND ORZO SOUP

Serves 4 / Serving Size: heaping 1 1/2 cups

The oregano-scented meatballs that star in this satisfying one-dish meal are extra moist and tasty thanks to the addition of a shredded carrot. Rice-shaped orzo pasta absorbs the flavors of the broth and cooks in just a few minutes. Adding the lemon juice at the end brightens the flavors. *(See photo insert.)*

Cooking spray

8 ounces 95% fat-free ground beef

1 medium carrot, finely shredded

1/4 cup plain dry whole-grain bread crumbs (lowest sodium available)

1 large egg white

1/2 teaspoon dried oregano, crumbled, divided use

1/2 teaspoon pepper, divided use

2 teaspoons olive oil

1 small onion, chopped

1 medium rib of celery, chopped

1 medium garlic clove, minced

3 cups fat-free, low-sodium chicken broth

1 (14.5-ounce) can no-salt-added diced tomatoes, undrained

2 tablespoons no-salt-added tomato paste

1/2 cup dried whole-wheat orzo

1 medium zucchini, chopped

2 teaspoons fresh lemon juice

1. Preheat the oven to 400°F. Lightly spray a broiler pan and rack with cooking spray. Set aside.

2. In a medium bowl, using your hands or a spoon, combine the beef, carrot, bread crumbs, egg white, 1/4 teaspoon oregano, and 1/4 teaspoon pepper. Shape into 32 meatballs. Arrange the meatballs in a single layer on the broiler rack.

3. Bake for 20 minutes, or until lightly browned on the outside and no longer pink in the center. Drain on paper towels.

4. Meanwhile, in a large saucepan, heat the oil over medium heat, swirling to coat the bottom. Cook the onion, celery, and garlic for 5 minutes, or until the onion is soft, stirring frequently.

5. Stir in the broth, tomatoes with liquid, tomato paste, and the remaining 1/4 teaspoon oregano and 1/4 teaspoon pepper. Increase the heat to high and bring to a boil. Stir in the orzo. Reduce the heat and simmer, covered, for 5 minutes.

6. Stir in the zucchini. Cook for 3 minutes, or until the orzo is tender and the zucchini is tender-crisp.

7. Gently stir in the meatballs. Cook for 1 minute. Remove from the heat. Stir in the lemon juice.

Exchanges / Choices
3 Vegetable, 1 Carbohydrate, 3 Lean Meat

Calories	290	Sodium	240 mg
Calories from Fat	80	Potassium	1010 mg
Total Fat	**9 g**	**Total Carbohydrate**	**33 g**
Saturated Fat	2.5 g	Dietary Fiber	5 g
Trans Fat	0 g	Sugars	11 g
Polyunsaturated Fat	1 g	**Protein**	**22 g**
Monounsaturated Fat	4.5 g	**Phosphorus**	**280 mg**
Cholesterol	**30 mg**		

HOME-STYLE VEGETABLE BEEF SOUP

Serves 8 / Serving Size: 1 1/2 cups

This hearty soup is bursting with garden-fresh vegetables and truly beefy flavor. It freezes well, so you may want to make a double batch to keep on hand for nights when you need a home-cooked meal in a hurry.

2 pounds boneless eye-of-round steak, all visible fat discarded, cut into 1/2-inch cubes

4 cups fat-free, low-sodium beef broth

2 cups water

1 (14.5-ounce) can no-salt-added diced tomatoes, undrained

1 pound red potatoes, cut into 3/4-inch cubes

2 medium carrots, cut into 1/2-inch slices

1 cup diced cauliflower

1 cup fresh, frozen, or no-salt-added canned whole-kernel corn, drained if canned

1 medium onion, diced

1 tablespoon Worcestershire sauce (lowest sodium available)

1 teaspoon dried thyme, crumbled

1 teaspoon dried oregano, crumbled

1/2 teaspoon salt

1/4 teaspoon pepper

Exchanges / Choices
1 Vegetable, 1 Starch, 3 Lean Meat

Calories	240	Sodium	260 mg
Calories from Fat	30	Potassium	1020 mg
Total Fat	3.5 g	Total Carbohydrate	21 g
Saturated Fat	1.5 g	Dietary Fiber	3 g
Trans Fat	0 g	Sugars	5 g
Polyunsaturated Fat	0.5 g	Protein	32 g
Monounsaturated Fat	1.5 g	Phosphorus	340 mg
Cholesterol	50 mg		

1. In a large stockpot or Dutch oven, stir together the beef, broth, water, and tomatoes with liquid. Bring to a boil over high heat. Reduce the heat and simmer, covered, for 45 minutes, or until the beef is just tender (no stirring needed).

2. Stir in the remaining ingredients. Simmer, covered, for 30 minutes, or until the vegetables and beef are tender, stirring occasionally.

PORK, BARLEY, AND VEGETABLE STEW

Serves 4 / Serving Size: 2 cups

A bowl of this stew will take away the chill during the winter months, but it's a nourishing meal year round. It packs in lean pork, chewy barley, and a variety of vegetables, including vitamin-rich greens.

6 cups fat-free, low-sodium chicken broth

1 pound boneless pork loin chops, all visible fat discarded, cut into 3/4-inch cubes

1 teaspoon ground cumin

1/4 teaspoon pepper

4 cups coarsely chopped collard greens or kale (about 1-inch pieces), any large stems discarded

1 cup baby carrots

1 cup frozen pearl onions

2 medium ribs of celery, cut into 1/2-inch slices

1/2 cup uncooked quick-cooking barley

2 medium garlic cloves, minced

Exchanges / Choices

1 Vegetable, 1 1/2 Starch, 3 Lean Meat

Calories	320	Sodium	300 mg
Calories from Fat	50	Potassium	1205 mg
Total Fat	**6 g**	**Total Carbohydrate**	**30 g**
Saturated Fat	1.5 g	Dietary Fiber	7 g
Trans Fat	0 g	Sugars	5 g
Polyunsaturated Fat	1 g	**Protein**	**32 g**
Monounsaturated Fat	2.5 g	Phosphorus	505 mg
Cholesterol	**70 mg**		

1. In a stockpot or Dutch oven, stir together the broth, pork, cumin, and pepper. Bring to a boil over high heat. Reduce the heat and simmer, covered, for 30 minutes, or until the pork is cooked through, stirring occasionally.

2. Stir in the remaining ingredients. Simmer, covered, for 30–35 minutes, or until the pork, vegetables, and barley are tender, stirring occasionally.

ITALIAN LENTIL SOUP

Serves 5 / Serving Size: 1 1/2 cups

Fresh zucchini and yellow summer squash add bright splashes of color to this sunny vegetarian soup, which tastes even better the next day when its Mediterranean flavors have had a chance to mingle. A last-minute sprinkle of Parmesan adds a toothsome touch.

1 teaspoon olive oil

1/2 cup diced onion

8 ounces sliced mushrooms, such as button, brown (cremini), portobello, or shiitake (stems discarded)

2 medium garlic cloves, minced

4 cups fat-free, low-sodium vegetable broth

1 (14.5-ounce) can no-salt-added tomatoes, undrained

1 cup dried lentils, sorted for stones and shriveled lentils, rinsed, and drained

1 teaspoon dried oregano, crumbled

1/4 teaspoon salt

1/4 teaspoon pepper

1 medium zucchini, diced

1 medium yellow summer squash, diced

1/4 cup plus 1 tablespoon shredded or grated Parmesan cheese

1. In a large saucepan, heat the oil over medium-high heat, swirling to coat the bottom. Cook the onion for 3 minutes, or until soft, stirring occasionally.

2. Stir in the mushrooms and garlic. Cook for 2–3 minutes, or until the mushrooms are tender, stirring occasionally.

3. Stir in the broth, tomatoes with liquid, lentils, oregano, salt, and pepper. Bring to a simmer, stirring occasionally. Reduce the heat and simmer, covered, for 30 minutes, or until the lentils are almost tender (no stirring needed).

4. Stir in the zucchini and yellow squash. Cook, covered, for 15 minutes, or until the lentils and vegetables are tender.

5. Just before serving, sprinkle the soup with the Parmesan.

Exchanges / Choices
2 Starch, 1 Vegetable, 1 Lean Meat

Calories	220	Sodium	210 mg
Calories from Fat	25	Potassium	1005 mg
Total Fat	**3 g**	**Total Carbohydrate**	**35 g**
Saturated Fat	1 g	Dietary Fiber	15 g
Trans Fat	0 g	Sugars	7 g
Polyunsaturated Fat	0.5 g	**Protein**	**15 g**
Monounsaturated Fat	1.5 g	Phosphorus	310 mg
Cholesterol	**<5 mg**		

MUSHROOM AND BARLEY STEW

Serves 4 / Serving Size: 1 1/2 cups

Chock-full of garden vegetables—carrot, parsnip, tomatoes, and bell pepper—and including three varieties of mushroom, this stew is intensely flavorful. The earthiness of barley adds richness and brings the stew together.

2/3 cup uncooked quick-cooking barley

2 teaspoons canola or corn oil

1 medium onion, chopped

1 medium carrot, chopped

1 small parsnip, peeled and chopped

1/2 small green, red, or yellow bell pepper, chopped

1 medium rib of celery, chopped

2 medium garlic cloves, crushed or minced

3 ounces button mushrooms, chopped

3 ounces brown (cremini) mushrooms, chopped

1 (14.5-ounce) can no-salt-added diced tomatoes, undrained

1 cup fat-free, low-sodium vegetable broth

1 cup water

1/4 ounce dried oyster or porcini mushrooms, chopped

1 tablespoon chopped fresh thyme or 1 teaspoon dried thyme, crumbled

1/4 teaspoon pepper

1/8 teaspoon salt

1. Prepare the barley using the package directions, omitting the salt. Drain well in a colander. Set aside.

2. Meanwhile, in a large saucepan, heat the oil over medium heat, swirling to coat the bottom. Cook the onion, carrot, parsnip, bell pepper, celery, and garlic for 8–10 minutes, or until the parsnip is tender, stirring occasionally.

3. Stir in the button and brown mushrooms. Cook for 2–4 minutes, or until they begin to soften, stirring occasionally.

4. Stir in the remaining ingredients. Increase the heat to high and bring to a boil. Stir in the barley. Reduce the heat and simmer, covered, for 10 minutes, stirring occasionally.

Cook's Tip on Parsnips: A good source of vitamin C, parsnips are root vegetables related to carrots. Buy parsnips that are 7–8 inches long. The larger ones are more likely to have woody cores and lack flavor. Store parsnips in perforated plastic bags in the crisper section of your refrigerator for up to three weeks. Parsnips are almost always eaten cooked, whether steamed, baked, boiled, or microwaved. Peel parsnips before cooking them.

Exchanges / Choices

2 Vegetable, 2 Carbohydrate

Calories	210	**Sodium**	120 mg
Calories from Fat	30	**Potassium**	830 mg
Total Fat	**3.5 g**	**Total Carbohydrate**	**40 g**
Saturated Fat	0.5 g	Dietary Fiber	10 g
Trans Fat	0 g	Sugars	8 g
Polyunsaturated Fat	1 g	**Protein**	**7 g**
Monounsaturated Fat	1.5 g	**Phosphorus**	**190 mg**
Cholesterol	**0 mg**		

VEGETABLE STEW WITH FRESH ROSEMARY

Serves 4 / Serving Size: 1 1/2 cups

This stew is like a farmers' market in a bowl with its wide range of colorful, tender vegetables, including green asparagus and zucchini, orange carrots, and bright yellow summer squash. If you have a green thumb, feel free to create new combinations based on your garden's bounty. *(See photo insert.)*

4 cups fat-free, low-sodium vegetable broth, divided use

8 small red potatoes, halved

1 cup baby carrots

1/2 cup frozen pearl onions

1 medium yellow summer squash, diced

1 small zucchini, diced

4 ounces sliced mushrooms, such as button, brown (cremini), portobello, or shiitake (stems discarded)

1 tablespoon chopped fresh rosemary or 1 teaspoon dried rosemary, crushed

1/4 teaspoon pepper

1/8 teaspoon salt

1/3 cup all-purpose flour

8 ounces asparagus, trimmed and cut diagonally into 1-inch pieces

2 tablespoons sliced green onions (green part only)

1/4 cup shredded or grated Parmesan cheese

1. In a large saucepan, bring 3 cups broth, the potatoes, carrots, and pearl onions to a simmer over medium-high heat. Reduce the heat and simmer, covered, for 15 minutes, or until the potatoes and carrots are tender.

2. Stir in the yellow squash, zucchini, mushrooms, rosemary, pepper, and salt.

Simmer, covered, for 3–4 minutes, or until both squashes are slightly tender.

3. In a medium bowl, whisk together the remaining 1 cup broth and the flour. Stir the flour mixture, asparagus, and green onions into the stew. Simmer for 2–3 minutes, or until the stew has thickened and the asparagus is tender-crisp.

4. Just before serving, sprinkle the stew with the Parmesan.

Cook's Tip: Some suggestions for substitutions include strips of bell pepper, cubed eggplant, cauliflower, broccoli, or corn instead of yellow summer squash; snow peas, sugar snap peas, baby spinach, or bok choy instead of asparagus; and fresh dill, oregano, basil, marjoram, thyme, or lemon thyme instead of rosemary.

Exchanges / Choices

2 Starch, 2 Vegetable

Calories	230	Sodium	310 mg
Calories from Fat	20	Potassium	1320 mg
Total Fat	**2 g**	**Total Carbohydrate**	**44 g**
Saturated Fat	1 g	Dietary Fiber	7 g
Trans Fat	0 g	Sugars	9 g
Polyunsaturated Fat	1 g	**Protein**	**9 g**
Monounsaturated Fat	1.5 g	**Phosphorus**	**240 mg**
Cholesterol	**<5 mg**		

| *Salads* |

Mixed Green Salad with Peppery Citrus Dressing 24
Salad Greens with Mixed-Herb Vinaigrette 25
Tomato Salad with Creamy Horseradish Dressing 26
Chopped Veggie Salad with Feta 27
Crunchy Asian Snow Pea Salad 28
Farmers' Market Veggie Salad 29
Fiesta Slaw 30
Italian Salsa Salad 31
Fanned Avocado Salad 32
Cantaloupe Wedges with Ginger-Citrus Sauce 33
Caribbean Fruit Salad Platter 34
Black Bean Cucumber Boats 35
Creamy Potato Salad 36
Tuna and Veggie Pasta Salad 37
Lemony Shrimp Salad 38
Chicken Antipasto Salad 39
Cranberry-Pecan Turkey Salad 40
Black Bean and Brown Rice Salad 41

MIXED GREEN SALAD WITH PEPPERY CITRUS DRESSING

Serves 5 / Serving Size: 1 1/2 cups salad and 2 tablespoons dressing

A double dose of citrus—from both grapefruit and lemon—provides a bright counterpoint to the heat of the jalapeño in this crisp salad. These lively flavors are a great way to wake up your taste buds at the start of your meal.

6 cups mixed salad greens

1 cup thinly sliced red onion

1 cup chopped fresh cilantro

Dressing

1 1/2 teaspoons grated grapefruit zest

1/2 cup fresh grapefruit juice

1 small fresh jalapeño, seeds and ribs discarded, minced

1 teaspoon grated lemon zest

1 1/2 tablespoons fresh lemon juice

1 1/2 teaspoons sugar

1 1/2 teaspoons canola or corn oil

1. Arrange the salad greens on a platter. Top with the onion and cilantro.

2. In a small bowl, whisk together the dressing ingredients. Pour over the salad, tossing gently to coat, or serve on the side.

Cook's Tip on Handling Hot Chiles: Hot chiles contain oils that can burn your skin, lips, and eyes. Wear plastic gloves or wash your hands thoroughly with warm, soapy water immediately after handling them.

Cook's Tip on Grapefruit: Grapefruit can interact with a number of medications, including many heart medicines. Be sure to check with your doctor or pharmacist if you take any medication, and substitute orange zest and fresh orange juice if necessary.

Exchanges / Choices

2 Vegetable

Calories	50	**Sodium**	10 mg
Calories from Fat	15	**Potassium**	250 mg
Total Fat	1.5 g	**Total Carbohydrate**	8 g
Saturated Fat	0 g	Dietary Fiber	2 g
Trans Fat	0 g	Sugars	5 g
Polyunsaturated Fat	0.5 g	**Protein**	1 g
Monounsaturated Fat	1 g	**Phosphorus**	30 mg
Cholesterol	0 mg		

SALAD GREENS WITH MIXED-HERB VINAIGRETTE

Serves 5 / Serving Size: 2 cups salad and 2 heaping tablespoons dressing

Delicate baby greens and an intensely flavored vinaigrette complement each other in this simple salad. The dressing is also very good on thin slices of vine-ripened tomato.

10 cups mixed baby salad greens

Dressing

1/3 cup finely chopped fresh basil or 1 1/2 table-spoons dried basil, crumbled

1/4 cup dry white wine (regular or nonalcoholic)

2 tablespoons chopped fresh oregano or 2 tea-spoons dried oregano, crumbled

2 tablespoons olive oil (extra virgin preferred)

1 teaspoon grated lemon zest

2 tablespoons fresh lemon juice

1 1/2 teaspoons cider vinegar

1 1/2 teaspoons Dijon mustard (lowest sodium available)

1 medium garlic clove, minced

1/4 teaspoon pepper

1/8 teaspoon salt

Exchanges / Choices
1 Vegetable, 1 Fat

Calories	80	**Sodium**	90 mg	
Calories from Fat	50	Potassium	295 mg	
Total Fat	**6 g**	**Total Carbohydrate**	**4 g**	
Saturated Fat	1 g	Dietary Fiber	2 g	
Trans Fat	0 g	Sugars	1 g	
Polyunsaturated Fat	1 g	**Protein**	**2 g**	
Monounsaturated Fat	4 g	**Phosphorus**	35 mg	
Cholesterol	**0 mg**			

1. Put the salad greens in a serving bowl.

2. In a small bowl, whisk together the dressing ingredients. Pour over the salad, tossing gently to coat.

TOMATO SALAD WITH CREAMY HORSERADISH DRESSING

Serves 4 / Serving Size: 1/2 cup greens, 3 tomato slices, and 2 tablespoons dressing

The sharpness of horseradish and the tang of Dijon mustard pair up in a thick, creamy dressing that lets the fresh, ripe tomatoes take a leading role. Mixed greens provide a crisp bed for the sweet, juicy tomatoes.

2 cups mixed salad greens

3 small tomatoes, each cut into 4 slices, or 12 ounces Italian plum (Roma) tomatoes, sliced or quartered

1/3 cup fat-free plain Greek yogurt

2 tablespoons light mayonnaise

1 teaspoon Dijon mustard (lowest sodium available)

1 teaspoon bottled white horseradish, drained

1/2 teaspoon pepper, divided use

1/16 teaspoon salt

Exchanges / Choices
1 Vegetable, 1/2 Fat

Calories	50	**Sodium**	130 mg
Calories from Fat	20	**Potassium**	320 mg
Total Fat	2 g	**Total Carbohydrate**	6 g
Saturated Fat	0 g	Dietary Fiber	2 g
Trans Fat	0 g	Sugars	4 g
Polyunsaturated Fat	1 g	**Protein**	3 g
Monounsaturated Fat	0.5 g	**Phosphorus**	60 mg
Cholesterol	<5 mg		

1. Place the salad greens on a platter. Arrange the tomatoes on top.

2. In a small bowl, whisk together the yogurt, mayonnaise, mustard, horseradish, 1/4 teaspoon pepper, and the salt.

3. Spoon the dressing onto the tomatoes or serve it on the side. Sprinkle with the remaining 1/4 teaspoon pepper.

Cook's Tip: The Creamy Horseradish Dressing also makes a great dip for fresh vegetables or a spread on sandwiches (try it with lean roast beef).

CHOPPED VEGGIE SALAD WITH FETA

Serves 4 / Serving Size: 3/4 cup

When you want a change from tossed green salad, try this easy alternative with a Greek flair. Tender artichoke hearts are combined with earthy mushrooms, juicy tomatoes, a variety of aromatic herbs, and tangy feta cheese. This salad is so full of flavor, you won't need any dressing!

1/2 (14-ounce) can quartered artichoke hearts, rinsed, drained, and coarsely chopped

4 ounces button mushrooms, chopped (about 1/4-inch cubes)

1 small tomato, seeded and chopped

1/4 cup finely chopped green onions

1/4 cup chopped fresh parsley

1 1/2 teaspoons dried basil, crumbled

3/4 teaspoon dried oregano, crumbled

1/2 ounce fat-free feta cheese with sun-dried tomatoes and basil, crumbled

Exchanges / Choices
2 Vegetable

Calories	50	**Sodium**	75 mg	
Calories from Fat	5	**Potassium**	360 mg	
Total Fat	0.5 g	**Total Carbohydrate**	9 g	
Saturated Fat	0 g	Dietary Fiber	6 g	
Trans Fat	0 g	Sugars	2 g	
Polyunsaturated Fat	0 g	**Protein**	3 g	
Monounsaturated Fat	0 g	**Phosphorus**	90 mg	
Cholesterol	<5 mg			

1. In a medium bowl, toss together all the ingredients except the feta.

2. Add the feta and toss gently. This salad is best if served within 1 hour.

Cook's Tip: Chopping the mushrooms into very small cubes allows them to absorb lots of flavor from the other ingredients.

CRUNCHY ASIAN SNOW PEA SALAD

Serves 4 / Serving Size: 1/2 cup

This crisp salad is just right with Asian entrées or as a change from coleslaw at picnics and barbecues. The delicate lemon-ginger dressing adds flavor without overpowering the crunchy vegetables. Try it with Sirloin and Broccoli Stir-Fry (page 100) or Asian Barbecued Pork Tenderloin (page 106).

Salad

1/2 (8-ounce) can sliced water chestnuts, rinsed, drained, and halved

1/2 cup finely chopped red onion

1/2 medium yellow bell pepper, finely chopped

3 ounces fresh snow peas (don't use frozen), trimmed and cut diagonally into 1/2-inch pieces

2 tablespoons chopped fresh cilantro

Dressing

2 tablespoons fresh lemon juice

1 1/2 teaspoons sugar

1 1/2 teaspoons canola or corn oil

1 teaspoon grated peeled gingerroot

1. In a medium bowl, stir together the salad ingredients.

2. In a small bowl, whisk together the dressing ingredients. Pour over the salad, tossing gently to coat.

Exchanges / Choices			
2 Vegetable			
Calories	60	**Sodium**	<5 mg
Calories from Fat	20	Potassium	160 mg
Total Fat	**2 g**	**Total Carbohydrate**	**10 g**
Saturated Fat	0 g	Dietary Fiber	2 g
Trans Fat	0 g	Sugars	5 g
Polyunsaturated Fat	0.5 g	**Protein**	**1 g**
Monounsaturated Fat	1 g	**Phosphorus**	**25 mg**
Cholesterol	**0 mg**		

FARMERS' MARKET VEGGIE SALAD

Serves 4 / Serving Size: 1/2 cup

Yellow bell pepper, orange carrot, green snow peas, and red onion make this salad as pleasing to the eye as it is to the palate. It's tossed with a sweet and tangy vinaigrette that allows the vegetables' freshness to shine.

Salad

1/2 medium yellow bell pepper, thinly sliced

1 small carrot, thinly sliced

1 ounce snow peas, trimmed

Dressing

1/4 cup thinly sliced red onion

2 1/4 teaspoons canola or corn oil

1 1/2 teaspoons sugar

1 1/2 teaspoons cider vinegar

1/8 teaspoon salt

Dash of red hot-pepper sauce, or to taste

1. In a medium bowl, stir together the salad ingredients.

2. In a small bowl, whisk together the dressing ingredients. Pour over the salad, tossing gently to coat.

Exchanges / Choices
1 Vegetable, 1/2 Fat

Calories	45	**Sodium**	65 mg
Calories from Fat	25	**Potassium**	125 mg
Total Fat	3 g	**Total Carbohydrate**	6 g
Saturated Fat	0 g	Dietary Fiber	1 g
Trans Fat	0 g	Sugars	3 g
Polyunsaturated Fat	1 g	**Protein**	1 g
Monounsaturated Fat	1.5 g	**Phosphorus**	20 mg
Cholesterol	0 mg		

FIESTA SLAW

Serves 5 / Serving Size: 1/2 cup

Although this vibrant coleslaw is good with almost any entrée, the blend of poblano pepper, cilantro, and lime juice makes it especially well suited to Mexican food. Try it with Fabulous Fajitas (page 94) or Tex-Mex Chicken Fingers (page 71).

Slaw

2 cups packaged shredded coleslaw mix

1/2 cup diced yellow summer squash

1/2 medium poblano pepper, seeds and ribs discarded, chopped

1/4 medium red bell pepper, chopped

1/4 cup chopped fresh cilantro

Dressing

1 1/2 tablespoons light mayonnaise

1 1/2 teaspoons sugar

1 1/2 teaspoons fresh lime juice

1/8 teaspoon salt

1. In a medium bowl, stir together the slaw ingredients.

2. In a small bowl, whisk together the dressing ingredients. Pour over the slaw, tossing gently to coat. Serve immediately for peak flavor.

Exchanges / Choices
2 Vegetable, 1/2 Fat

Calories	60	Sodium	85 mg
Calories from Fat	25	Potassium	175 mg
Total Fat	2.5 g	Total Carbohydrate	10 g
Saturated Fat	0 g	Dietary Fiber	1 g
Trans Fat	0 g	Sugars	2 g
Polyunsaturated Fat	1 g	Protein	1 g
Monounsaturated Fat	0.5 g	Phosphorus	25 mg
Cholesterol	<5 mg		

ITALIAN SALSA SALAD

Serves 6 / Serving Size: 1/2 cup

This Italian-inspired salsa is bursting with flavor from grape tomatoes, bell pepper, red onion, capers, and a variety of herbs. Crushed red pepper flakes add a small flash of heat. Use this chunky salad to dress up grilled fish or chicken, or serve atop whole-grain pasta instead of sauce.

10 ounces grape tomatoes or cherry tomatoes, halved (about 2 cups)

1/2 medium green bell pepper, chopped

1/2 cup chopped red onion

1/2 cup chopped fresh parsley

2 tablespoons capers, rinsed and drained

2 tablespoons cider vinegar

1 tablespoon olive oil (extra virgin preferred)

2 teaspoons dried basil, crumbled

1 teaspoon dried oregano, crumbled

1/8 teaspoon crushed red pepper flakes

1/8 teaspoon salt

Exchanges / Choices
1 Vegetable, 1/2 Fat

Calories	40	**Sodium**	120 mg
Calories from Fat	25	**Potassium**	190 mg
Total Fat	2.5 g	**Total Carbohydrate**	4 g
Saturated Fat	0 g	Dietary Fiber	1 g
Trans Fat	0 g	Sugars	2 g
Polyunsaturated Fat	0.5 g	**Protein**	1 g
Monounsaturated Fat	2 g	**Phosphorus**	20 mg
Cholesterol	0 mg		

1. In a medium bowl, gently toss together all the ingredients. Let stand for 10 minutes before serving.

Cook's Tip: A variety of cherry tomato, the grape tomato is sweet and less watery than its relative. That means it won't dilute the flavor of other ingredients with which it's combined.

FANNED AVOCADO SALAD

Serves 6 / Serving Size: 1/2 cup

Earthy spinach, crunchy cucumber, fragrant tomatoes, and sharp feta complement the creamy richness of avocado in this attractive salad. A slightly spicy lemon-lime
dressing takes it from simple to sensational. *(See photo insert.)*

Dressing

2 tablespoons fresh lime juice

2 tablespoons fresh lemon juice

1/4 teaspoon pepper

1/4 teaspoon red hot-pepper sauce

1/8 teaspoon salt

Salad

18 medium spinach leaves

1/2 medium cucumber, peeled and sliced

1 medium tomato, sliced crosswise and halved

1 medium avocado, thinly sliced

1/2 cup chopped fresh cilantro

1 ounce fat-free feta cheese, crumbled

1. In a small bowl, whisk together the dressing ingredients.

2. On a platter, decoratively arrange the spinach, cucumber, tomato, and avocado like a fan or an accordion. Pour the dressing over all. Sprinkle with the cilantro and feta. Serve immediately for peak flavor and so the spinach doesn't wilt.

Exchanges / Choices

1 Vegetable, 1 Fat

Calories	70	Sodium	160 mg
Calories from Fat	30	Potassium	365 mg
Total Fat	**3.5 g**	**Total Carbohydrate**	**5 g**
Saturated Fat	0.5 g	Dietary Fiber	3 g
Trans Fat	0 g	Sugars	2 g
Polyunsaturated Fat	0.5 g	**Protein**	**3 g**
Monounsaturated Fat	2 g	**Phosphorus**	**55 mg**
Cholesterol	**<5 mg**		

CANTALOUPE WEDGES WITH GINGER-CITRUS SAUCE

**Serves 4 / Serving Size: 2 cantaloupe wedges,
2 tablespoons blueberries, and 2 tablespoons sauce**

Cantaloupe and blueberries make a perfect pair, and a zesty citrus sauce emphasizes their natural sweetness. This versatile fruit salad is great for breakfast or brunch, and can even be served as a light dessert.

Sauce

1/4 cup frozen 100% orange juice concentrate

1 teaspoon grated lemon zest

2 tablespoons fresh lemon juice

1 1/2 tablespoons honey

1 teaspoon grated peeled gingerroot

---

1 medium cantaloupe (about 1 pound), peeled, seeded, and cut into 8 wedges or diced

1/2 cup blueberries

Exchanges / Choices			
2 Fruit			
Calories	100	**Sodium**	20 mg
Calories from Fat	0	**Potassium**	450 mg
Total Fat	**0 g**	**Total Carbohydrate**	**26 g**
Saturated Fat	0 g	Dietary Fiber	2 g
Trans Fat	0 g	Sugars	24 g
Polyunsaturated Fat	0 g	**Protein**	**2 g**
Monounsaturated Fat	0 g	**Phosphorus**	**30 mg**
Cholesterol	**0 mg**		

1. In a small bowl, whisk together the sauce ingredients.

2. Arrange the cantaloupe on plates. Sprinkle with the blueberries. Spoon the sauce over the fruit. Serve immediately for peak flavor.

CARIBBEAN FRUIT SALAD PLATTER

Serves 12 / Serving Size: 1/2 cup

This refreshing tropical fruit platter is like an island vacation on a plate.
Creamy banana is combined with juicy strawberries, mango, and kiwifruit, and then lightly dressed with citrus before being topped off with crunchy toasted coconut. It's the perfect dish to serve at a barbecue, but it's also easy to reduce the amounts if you want to make fewer servings.

2 cups quartered hulled strawberries

1 medium mango, cubed

1 medium banana, sliced diagonally

2 medium kiwifruit, peeled and cut into wedges

1 teaspoon grated orange zest

Juice of 1 medium orange

1 teaspoon grated lemon zest

1 tablespoon fresh lemon juice

1 1/2 teaspoons sugar

1/2 cup sweetened flaked coconut, toasted

Exchanges / Choices			
1 Fruit			
Calories	50	**Sodium**	10 mg
Calories from Fat	10	**Potassium**	170 mg
Total Fat	1 g	**Total Carbohydrate**	12 g
Saturated Fat	1 g	Dietary Fiber	2 g
Trans Fat	0 g	Sugars	8 g
Polyunsaturated Fat	0 g	**Protein**	1 g
Monounsaturated Fat	0 g	**Phosphorus**	20 mg
Cholesterol	0 mg		

1. Arrange the strawberries, mango, banana, and kiwifruit on a platter.

2. In a small bowl, whisk together the remaining ingredients except the coconut. Pour the orange juice mixture over the fruit. Sprinkle with the coconut.

BLACK BEAN CUCUMBER BOATS

Serves 4 / Serving Size: 1 stuffed cucumber half

Crisp, cool cucumber halves make an excellent edible vessel for a savory, lightly dressed mixture of black beans, sweet red onion, and mild Anaheim pepper. Try this with Southwestern Pork Tenderloin Skillet (page 107).

2 large cucumbers, halved lengthwise

1/2 (15.5-ounce) can no-salt-added black beans, rinsed and drained

1 medium Anaheim pepper, seeds and ribs discarded, finely chopped

1/3 cup finely chopped red onion

1/4 cup chopped fresh cilantro

2 tablespoons cider vinegar

2 tablespoons fresh lime juice

1/8 teaspoon salt

1 tablespoon olive oil (extra virgin preferred)

Exchanges / Choices

1 Carbohydrate, 1 Fat

Calories	120	Sodium	60 mg
Calories from Fat	35	Potassium	450 mg
Total Fat	**4 g**	**Total Carbohydrate**	**17 g**
Saturated Fat	0.5 g	Dietary Fiber	4 g
Trans Fat	0 g	Sugars	4 g
Polyunsaturated Fat	0.5 g	**Protein**	**5 g**
Monounsaturated Fat	2.5 g	**Phosphorus**	**95 mg**
Cholesterol	**0 mg**		

1. Using a spoon, remove and discard the cucumber seeds. Carefully scoop out and keep most of the flesh of the cucumber, leaving a thin shell. Chop the cucumber flesh.

2. In a medium bowl, toss together the chopped cucumber and the remaining ingredients except the oil. Gently stir in the oil.

3. Spoon the bean mixture into each cucumber half.

Cook's Tip: You can prepare the cucumber boats up to 24 hours in advance; however, it's better to wait until serving time to assemble the bean stuffing.

CREAMY POTATO SALAD

Serves 4 / Serving Size: 1/2 cup

Flecks of red and green bell pepper brighten up this zippy potato salad, which gets its zing from dry mustard and cider vinegar. Double or triple the recipe if you want to feed a crowd.

8 ounces red potatoes, cut into 1/2-inch cubes

1/2 medium green bell pepper, finely chopped

1/2 medium rib of celery, finely chopped

3 tablespoons finely chopped red onion

1 1/2 tablespoons light mayonnaise

1 tablespoon fat-free sour cream

2 1/4 teaspoons cider vinegar

1 teaspoon dry mustard

1/8 teaspoon salt

Exchanges / Choices
1 Carbohydrate

Calories	70	Sodium	105 mg
Calories from Fat	20	Potassium	325 mg
Total Fat	**2 g**	**Total Carbohydrate**	**11 g**
Saturated Fat	0 g	Dietary Fiber	1 g
Trans Fat	0 g	Sugars	2 g
Polyunsaturated Fat	1 g	**Protein**	**2 g**
Monounsaturated Fat	0.5 g	**Phosphorus**	**45 mg**
Cholesterol	**0 mg**		

1. In a medium saucepan, steam the potatoes for 8–10 minutes, or until tender. Transfer to a colander and rinse with cold water to cool completely. Shake off the excess liquid.

2. Meanwhile, in a medium bowl, stir together the remaining ingredients.

3. Stir the potatoes into the bell pepper mixture. Cover and refrigerate for 30 minutes.

TUNA AND VEGGIE PASTA SALAD

Serves 4 / Serving Size: 1 1/2 cups

This fresh take on tuna salad combines the fish with whole-grain pasta, fresh veggies, grape tomatoes, creamy light mayonnaise, and a balsamic vinaigrette. Serve it on its own or over fresh mixed salad greens.

6 ounces dried whole-grain rotini

2 (5-ounce) cans very low sodium chunk white albacore tuna, drained and flaked

6 ounces grape tomatoes, chopped

1/2 small cucumber, chopped

1/2 medium red bell pepper, chopped

1/3 small sweet onion, such as Vidalia, Maui, or Oso Sweet, chopped

1/4 cup light balsamic vinaigrette (lowest sodium available)

1/4 cup light mayonnaise

2 tablespoons chopped fresh cilantro

Exchanges / Choices
2 1/2 Starch, 1 Vegetable, 2 Lean Meat

Calories	310	Sodium	280 mg
Calories from Fat	60	Potassium	490 mg
Total Fat	**7 g**	**Total Carbohydrate**	**41 g**
Saturated Fat	1 g	Dietary Fiber	5 g
Trans Fat	0 g	Sugars	7 g
Polyunsaturated Fat	3 g	**Protein**	**24 g**
Monounsaturated Fat	1.5 g	**Phosphorus**	**300 mg**
Cholesterol	**30 mg**		

1. Prepare the pasta using the package directions, omitting the salt. Transfer to a colander. Rinse with cold water to cool completely. Drain well. Transfer to a large bowl.

2. Gently stir in the remaining ingredients. Serve immediately or cover and refrigerate for up to 24 hours.

LEMONY SHRIMP SALAD

Serves 4 / Serving Size: 1 cup salad greens and 3/4 cup shrimp mixture

A triple hit of lemon—zest, juice, and wedges—complements a triple hit of spiciness—Creole seasoning, black pepper, and red hot-pepper sauce—in this entrée salad.

10 ounces peeled raw medium shrimp, rinsed and patted dry

2 large hard-boiled eggs

1/2 cup finely chopped green onions

1/2 cup finely chopped celery

1/4 cup chopped fresh parsley

1 teaspoon grated lemon zest

1/4 cup fresh lemon juice

2 tablespoons fat-free sour cream

2 tablespoons light mayonnaise

1/2 teaspoon salt-free Creole or Cajun seasoning blend

1/4 teaspoon pepper

1/8 teaspoon red hot-pepper sauce

4 cups mixed salad greens

2 medium lemons, each cut into 4 wedges

1. In a large saucepan, bring 6 cups of water to a boil over high heat. Boil the shrimp for 3 minutes, or until pink on the outside. Transfer to a colander. Rinse with cold water to cool completely. Drain well on paper towels.

2. Meanwhile, cut each egg in half. Discard 2 yolk halves. Chop the remaining 2 yolk halves and all the whites.

3. In a medium bowl, stir together the green onions, celery, parsley, lemon zest, lemon juice, sour cream, mayonnaise, seasoning blend, pepper, and hot-pepper sauce. Add the shrimp and toss gently. Add the eggs and toss gently.

4. Place the salad greens on plates. Top each salad with the shrimp mixture. Serve with the lemon wedges.

Cook's Tip on Creole or Cajun Seasoning Blend: To make your own salt-free Creole or Cajun seasoning blend, stir together 1 tablespoon each of chili powder, ground cumin, garlic powder, onion powder, and paprika, plus 2 teaspoons ground oregano, 2 teaspoons ground thyme, and 1/2 teaspoon pepper. Store the mixture in an airtight container at room temperature for up to six months.

Exchanges / Choices
2 Vegetable, 2 Lean Meat

Calories	130	Sodium	520 mg
Calories from Fat	35	Potassium	430 mg
Total Fat	4 g	Total Carbohydrate	13 g
Saturated Fat	1 g	Dietary Fiber	4 g
Trans Fat	0 g	Sugars	3 g
Polyunsaturated Fat	1.5 g	Protein	14 g
Monounsaturated Fat	1 g	Phosphorus	240 mg
Cholesterol	140 mg		

CHICKEN ANTIPASTO SALAD

Serves 4 / Serving Size: heaping 1 1/2 cups

This filling salad has all the flavors of a traditional antipasto platter, but with a heart-healthy twist. Ingredients such as turkey pepperoni and fat-free feta cheese are so flavorful that just a little bit goes a long way.

3 ounces dried whole-grain rotini

12 ounces frozen artichoke hearts, thawed and coarsley chopped

8 ounces boneless, skinless chicken breasts, cooked without salt, diced

1 medium green bell pepper, finely chopped

8 slices turkey pepperoni, chopped

1/2 cup thinly sliced red onion

1/3 cup chopped roasted red bell peppers, drained if bottled

1 1/2 teaspoons dried basil, crumbled

1 tablespoon cider vinegar

1 tablespoon olive oil (extra virgin preferred)

1 ounce fat-free feta cheese with sun-dried tomato and basil, crumbled

Cook's Tip: To make this salad ahead, stir together all the ingredients except the vinegar, oil, and feta. Cover and refrigerate until needed. Just before serving, add the vinegar and oil and toss gently. Add the feta and toss gently.

Exchanges / Choices
3 Vegetable, 1 Starch, 3 Lean Meat

Calories	280	Sodium	400 mg
Calories from Fat	60	Potassium	560 mg
Total Fat	**7 g**	**Total Carbohydrate**	**30 g**
Saturated Fat	1.5 g	Dietary Fiber	10 g
Trans Fat	0 g	Sugars	4 g
Polyunsaturated Fat	1 g	**Protein**	**26 g**
Monounsaturated Fat	4 g	**Phosphorus**	**285 mg**
Cholesterol	**55 mg**		

1. Prepare the pasta using the package directions, omitting the salt. Transfer to a colander. Rinse with cold water to cool completely. Drain well.

2. Meanwhile, in a large bowl, stir together the artichokes, chicken, bell pepper, pepperoni, onion, roasted peppers, and basil.

3. Add the pasta, vinegar, and oil to the artichoke mixture and toss gently. Add the feta and toss gently. Serve immediately for peak flavor.

CRANBERRY-PECAN TURKEY SALAD

Serves 4 / Serving Size: heaping 3/4 cup turkey mixture and 1/2 medium apple

This so-simple salad, which combines turkey breast with creamy yogurt, tart cranberries, and crunchy pecans, is especially good with leftovers from Roast Turkey with Orange-Spice Rub (page 83). Spread the salad over the accompanying apple slices for a crisp open-face "sandwich."

1/4 cup fat-free vanilla yogurt

2 tablespoons light mayonnaise

12 ounces boneless, skinless cooked turkey breast, cooked without salt, diced (about 2 1/2 cups)

1/2 cup sweetened dried cranberries

1 medium rib of celery, sliced

1/4 cup finely chopped red onion

1 ounce pecan chips, dry-roasted

2 medium apples, sliced

Exchanges / Choices
2 Fruit, 4 Lean Meat

Calories	310	Sodium	110 mg
Calories from Fat	80	Potassium	490 mg
Total Fat	**9 g**	**Total Carbohydrate**	**30 g**
Saturated Fat	1.5 g	Dietary Fiber	4 g
Trans Fat	0 g	Sugars	23 g
Polyunsaturated Fat	3 g	**Protein**	**27 g**
Monounsaturated Fat	4 g	**Phosphorus**	**260 mg**
Cholesterol	**70 mg**		

1. In a medium bowl, whisk together the yogurt and mayonnaise.

2. Stir in the remaining ingredients except the apples.

3. Fan the apples in a half-circle on each of four plates. Spoon the turkey mixture beside the apple slices.

BLACK BEAN AND BROWN RICE SALAD

Serves 4 / Serving Size: 1 1/2 cups

Avocado adds a smooth richness to this Mexican-inspired entrée salad that can be ready at a moment's notice. Tender, mild black beans are an excellent meatless source of protein.

1 (10-ounce) package frozen brown rice

1 (15.5-ounce) can no-salt-added black beans, rinsed and drained

1 medium avocado, chopped

1 medium tomato, diced

4 medium green onions, chopped

6–7 sprigs of fresh cilantro, chopped

2 tablespoons fresh lime juice

2 teaspoons olive oil (extra virgin preferred)

1/4–1/2 teaspoon red hot-pepper sauce, or to taste

1/4 teaspoon salt

1. Prepare the rice using the package directions. Spread in a thin layer on a baking sheet to cool quickly (about 10 minutes).

2. Meanwhile, in a large bowl, gently stir together the beans, avocado, tomato, green onions, and cilantro. Gently stir in the lime juice, oil, hot-pepper sauce, and salt.

3. Gently stir in the cooled rice. Serve immediately for peak flavor and texture or cover and refrigerate for up to 4 hours.

Cook's Tip: Frozen brown rice is already cooked and has no added sodium or fat. After just a few minutes in the microwave or on top of the stove, it's ready to use. When you want a change of flavor, substitute barley, bulgur, whole-grain pasta, or any other whole grain for the brown rice in this very versatile salad.

Exchanges / Choices
2 Starch, 1 Vegetable, 2 Fat

Calories	260	**Sodium**	140 mg
Calories from Fat	80	**Potassium**	605 mg
Total Fat	**9 g**	**Total Carbohydrate**	**38 g**
Saturated Fat	1 g	Dietary Fiber	10 g
Trans Fat	0 g	Sugars	2 g
Polyunsaturated Fat	1 g	**Protein**	**9 g**
Monounsaturated Fat	5 g	**Phosphorus**	175 mg
Cholesterol	**0 mg**		

| *Seafood* |

BAKED FISH STICKS WITH A KICK

Serves 4 / Serving Size: 3 ounces fish

These fish sticks are all grown up, with tang from buttermilk, yogurt, and lemon juice, plus zip from horseradish, Dijon mustard, and pepper. With such a flavorful coating, no sauce is needed. Try them with roasted vegetables and baked sweet potato fries.

Cooking spray

1/4 cup low-fat buttermilk

1/4 cup fat-free plain yogurt

2 tablespoons fresh lemon juice

1 tablespoon bottled white horseradish, drained

1 teaspoon Dijon mustard (lowest sodium available)

1/2 teaspoon dried thyme, crumbled

1/4 teaspoon pepper

1/3 cup finely crushed whole-grain crispbread (lowest sodium available)

1/4 cup yellow cornmeal

1 pound cod, orange roughy, or other firm white fish fillets, rinsed, patted dry, and cut crosswise into 3/4-inch strips

1. Preheat the oven to 475°F. Lightly spray a baking sheet with cooking spray.

2. In a medium shallow dish, whisk together the buttermilk, yogurt, lemon juice, horseradish, mustard, thyme, and pepper. In a separate medium shallow dish, stir together the crispbread crumbs and cornmeal. Put the dishes and baking sheet in a row, assembly-line fashion. Dip the fish in the buttermilk mixture, then in the crispbread mixture, turning to coat at each step and gently shaking off any excess. Using your fingertips, gently press the coating mixture so it adheres to the fish.

3. Arrange the fish in a single layer on the baking sheet. Lightly spray the top of the fish with cooking spray.

4. Bake for 12–15 minutes, or until the fish flakes easily when tested with a fork and the top coating is crisp and golden.

Cook's Tip: It is easier to cut the fish into even-sized sticks when the fish is very cold or slightly frozen.

Exchanges / Choices
1 1/2 Starch, 2 Lean Meat

Calories	220	**Sodium**	225 mg
Calories from Fat	20	**Potassium**	640 mg
Total Fat	2 g	**Total Carbohydrate**	27 g
Saturated Fat	0.5 g	Dietary Fiber	4 g
Trans Fat	0 g	Sugars	3 g
Polyunsaturated Fat	0.5 g	**Protein**	24 g
Monounsaturated Fat	0.5 g	**Phosphorus**	345 mg
Cholesterol	50 mg		

BAKED FISH FILLETS WITH THYME-DIJON TOPPING

Serves 4 / Serving Size: 3 ounces fish and 1 tablespoon topping

This dish features baked fish fillets topped with a simple but sophisticated blend of margarine, mustard, and herbs. Keep the sides equally simple with Lemon-Mint Sugar Snaps (page 146) or Green Beans with Mushrooms and Onions (page 136).

Cooking spray

4 grouper or other mild fish fillets (about 4 ounces each), rinsed and patted dry

3 tablespoons light tub margarine

2 tablespoons finely chopped fresh parsley

1 teaspoon Dijon mustard (lowest sodium available)

1/4 teaspoon dried thyme, crumbled

1/4 teaspoon red hot-pepper sauce

1/8 teaspoon salt

Exchanges / Choices			
3 Lean Meat			
Calories	140	**Sodium**	210 mg
Calories from Fat	45	**Potassium**	565 mg
Total Fat	5 g	**Total Carbohydrate**	0 g
Saturated Fat	1 g	Dietary Fiber	0 g
Trans Fat	0 g	Sugars	0 g
Polyunsaturated Fat	1.5 g	**Protein**	22 g
Monounsaturated Fat	1.5 g	**Phosphorus**	185 mg
Cholesterol	40 mg		

1. Preheat the oven to 350°F. Lightly spray a baking sheet with cooking spray.

2. Place the fish on the baking sheet. Bake for 18–20 minutes, or until the fish flakes easily when tested with a fork.

3. Meanwhile, in a small bowl, stir together the remaining ingredients.

4. Spread the margarine mixture over the fish.

CORNMEAL-COATED CATFISH WITH TOMATO SAUCE

Serves 4 / Serving Size: 3 ounces fish and 2 tablespoons sauce

Catfish with a hint of orange in its crisp cornmeal coating partners well with oregano-infused tomato sauce that takes just minutes to prepare.

Sauce

1 teaspoon olive oil

1 small onion, chopped

2 tablespoons grated carrot

1 medium garlic clove, minced

1 (8-ounce) can no-salt-added tomato sauce

2 tablespoons chopped fresh parsley

1/2 teaspoon dried oregano, crumbled

1/4 teaspoon crushed red pepper flakes

Cooking spray

1/3 cup low-fat buttermilk

1 teaspoon grated orange zest

1 tablespoon fresh orange juice

1/2 cup yellow cornmeal

1 medium Anaheim pepper, seeds and ribs discarded, finely chopped

1/4 teaspoon salt

4 catfish fillets (4 ounces each), rinsed and patted dry

1. In a medium nonstick skillet, heat the oil over medium heat, swirling to coat the bottom. Cook the onion, carrot, and garlic for 3 minutes, or until the onion is soft.

2. Stir in the remaining sauce ingredients. Increase the heat to medium high and bring to a boil. Reduce the heat and simmer, partially covered, for 20 minutes.

3. Meanwhile, preheat the oven to 450°F. Lightly spray an 11 x 7 x 2-inch baking dish with cooking spray.

4. In a medium shallow dish, whisk together the buttermilk and orange juice. In a separate medium shallow dish, stir together the orange zest, cornmeal, Anaheim pepper, and salt. Set the dishes and baking dish in a row, assembly-line fashion. Dip the fish in the buttermilk mixture, then in the cornmeal mixture, turning to coat at each step and gently shaking off any excess. Using your fingertips, gently press the coating mixture so it adheres to the fish.

5. Arrange the fish in a single layer in the baking dish. Lightly spray the top of the fish with cooking spray.

6. Bake for 12–15 minutes, or until the top coating is slightly crisp and the fish flakes easily when tested with a fork.

7. Spoon the sauce over the fish.

Exchanges / Choices	
1 Starch, 2 Vegetable, 2 Lean Meat	

Calories	230	**Sodium**	190 mg
Calories from Fat	50	**Potassium**	835 mg
Total Fat	6 g	**Total Carbohydrate**	24 g
Saturated Fat	1 g	Dietary Fiber	3 g
Trans Fat	0 g	Sugars	7 g
Polyunsaturated Fat	1.5 g	**Protein**	22 g
Monounsaturated Fat	2 g	**Phosphorus**	330 mg
Cholesterol	70 mg		

PAN-FRIED CATFISH WITH FRESH VEGGIE RELISH

Serves 4 / Serving Size: 3 ounces fish and 1/4 cup relish

Crisp, flavor-packed vegetables make this relish a cooling accompaniment to the spicy fish, while fresh lemon juice and gingerroot add zing.

Relish

1 medium red bell pepper, very finely chopped

1 cup very finely chopped carrots

2 tablespoons very finely chopped red onion

2 tablespoons fresh lemon juice

1 1/2 teaspoons sugar

3/4 teaspoon grated peeled gingerroot

1/2 teaspoon chili powder

1/2 teaspoon dried oregano, crumbled

1/4 teaspoon salt

1/4 teaspoon pepper

4 catfish fillets (about 4 ounces each), rinsed and patted dry

2 teaspoons canola or corn oil

Exchanges / Choices
2 Vegetable, 2 Lean Meat

Calories	160	**Sodium**	180 mg
Calories from Fat	50	**Potassium**	590 mg
Total Fat	6 g	**Total Carbohydrate**	8 g
Saturated Fat	1 g	Dietary Fiber	2 g
Trans Fat	0 g	Sugars	5 g
Polyunsaturated Fat	1.5 g	**Protein**	19 g
Monounsaturated Fat	2.5 g	**Phosphorus**	260 mg
Cholesterol	70 mg		

1. In a medium bowl, stir together the relish ingredients. Set aside.

2. In a small bowl, stir together the chili powder, oregano, salt, and pepper. Sprinkle over the fish. Using your fingertips, gently press the mixture so it adheres to the fish.

3. In a large nonstick skillet, heat the oil over medium-high heat, swirling to coat the bottom. Cook the fish for 3 minutes. Turn over. Cook for 3 minutes, or until the fish flakes easily when tested with a fork.

4. Serve the fish with the relish spooned on top or on the side.

OVEN-FRIED HADDOCK SANDWICH

Serves 4 / Serving Size: 1 sandwich

Cracker-coated haddock fillets are layered with tomato, lettuce, and creamy home-made tartar sauce in these delicious sandwiches. *(See photo insert.)*

Fish

Cooking spray

1/3 cup fat-free evaporated milk

1 teaspoon grated lemon zest

2 tablespoons fresh lemon juice

1 tablespoon bottled white horseradish, drained

1/3 cup finely crushed whole-grain crispbread (lowest sodium available)

1/4 cup yellow cornmeal

1/4 teaspoon crushed red pepper flakes

1 pound haddock or other mild fish fillets, such as cod or flounder, rinsed and patted dry

Tartar Sauce

2 tablespoons light mayonnaise

1 teaspoon minced red onion

1 teaspoon minced fresh Italian (flat-leaf) parsley

1 teaspoon minced sweet pickle or cornichon

4 whole-grain round sandwich thins (lowest sodium available), halved and toasted

4 medium-large lettuce leaves, any variety

8 slices tomato

1. Preheat the oven to 450°F. Lightly spray a baking sheet with cooking spray.

2. In a shallow glass bowl, whisk together the evaporated milk, lemon zest, lemon juice, and horseradish. In a separate shallow bowl, stir together the crispbread, cornmeal, and red pepper flakes. Set the dishes and baking sheet in a row, assembly-line fashion. Dip the fish in the milk mixture, then in the crispbread mixture, turning to coat at each step and gently shaking off any excess. Using your fingertips, gently press the mixture so it adheres to the fish.

3. Place the fish on the baking sheet. Lightly spray the top of the fish with cooking spray.

4. Bake for 12–14 minutes, or until the fish flakes easily when tested with a fork.

5. Meanwhile, in a small bowl, stir together the tartar sauce ingredients.

6. To assemble the sandwiches, spread the tartar sauce on the inside of the tops of the sandwich thins. Layer the fish, lettuce, and tomato slices on the bottoms of the sandwich thins. Put the top on each sandwich.

Cook's Tip: If you can't find whole-grain crispbread, substitute fat-free, unsalted whole-grain crackers.

Exchanges / Choices
2 Starch, 1 Vegetable, 3 Lean Meat

Calories	310	Sodium	520 mg
Calories from Fat	35	Potassium	690 mg
Total Fat	**4 g**	**Total Carbohydrate**	**44 g**
Saturated Fat	1 g	Dietary Fiber	9 g
Trans Fat	0 g	Sugars	6 g
Polyunsaturated Fat	1.5 g	**Protein**	**28 g**
Monounsaturated Fat	1 g	**Phosphorus**	**406 mg**
Cholesterol	**40 mg**		

CREOLE-SAUCED HALIBUT

Serves 4 / Serving Size: 3 ounces fish and 1/2 cup sauce

Tender baked fish fillets are topped with a sauce that starts with the "holy trinity" of onion, celery, and bell pepper, then builds flavor with the addition of tomatoes, green onions, capers, and a touch of hot-pepper sauce. Serve this with brown or wild rice and a southern-flavored side, such as Down-Home Greens (page 138).

Cooking spray

4 halibut fillets with skin (about 5 ounces each), rinsed and patted dry

1 large onion, chopped

1 medium green bell pepper, chopped

1 1/2 medium ribs of celery, chopped

1 teaspoon dried thyme, crumbled

1 medium garlic clove, minced

1 cup diced grape tomatoes or cherry tomatoes

1/4 cup finely chopped green onions

2 tablespoons capers, drained

1/4 cup chopped fresh parsley

2 tablespoons light tub margarine

1/2 teaspoon red hot-pepper sauce, or to taste

1/4 teaspoon salt

1. Preheat the oven to 400°F. Lightly spray a baking sheet with cooking spray.

2. Place the fish with the skin side down on the baking sheet. Bake for 18–20 minutes, or until the fish flakes easily when tested with a fork.

3. Meanwhile, lightly spray a large skillet with cooking spray. Cook the onion, bell pepper, celery, thyme, and garlic over medium-high heat for 3 minutes, or until the onion is soft, stirring occasionally.

4. Stir the tomatoes, green onions, and capers into the bell pepper mixture. Cook for 2 minutes, or until the tomatoes are soft, stirring constantly. Remove from the heat.

5. Stir in the remaining ingredients. Cover to keep warm.

6. When the fish is cooked, transfer it to serving plates. Spoon the bell pepper mixture over the fish.

Exchanges / Choices
2 Vegetable, 4 Lean Meat

Calories	220	Sodium	410 mg
Calories from Fat	60	Potassium	950 mg
Total Fat	**7 g**	**Total Carbohydrate**	**11 g**
Saturated Fat	1.5 g	Dietary Fiber	3 g
Trans Fat	0 g	Sugars	4 g
Polyunsaturated Fat	2.5 g	**Protein**	**31 g**
Monounsaturated Fat	2.5 g	**Phosphorus**	**385 mg**
Cholesterol	**100 mg**		

ROASTED CUMIN HALIBUT AND FRESH ORANGE SALSA

Serves 4 / Serving Size: 3 ounces fish and 1/3 cup salsa

Spicy citrus salsa perks up flaky baked fish and goes well with chicken and pork, too. The spicy jalapeño is a perfect counterpoint to the sweet, juicy fruit, while the radishes add crunch and a bit more bite.

Cooking spray

4 halibut or other mild fish fillets with skin (about 5 ounces each), rinsed and patted dry

2 teaspoons ground cumin

1 teaspoon paprika

1/4 teaspoon salt

Salsa

1 medium orange, peeled and cut into 1/2-inch pieces (about 1 cup) or 1 cup pineapple chunks

1 small fresh jalapeño, seeds and ribs discarded, minced

1/4 cup finely chopped radishes

1/4 cup chopped fresh cilantro

2 tablespoons fresh lemon juice

1 teaspoon sugar

1 teaspoon grated peeled gingerroot

1. Preheat the oven to 350°F. Lightly spray a baking sheet with cooking spray.

2. Place the fish with the skin side down on the baking sheet.

3. In a small bowl, stir together the cumin, paprika, and salt. Sprinkle over the flesh side of the fish. Lightly spray with cooking spray.

4. Bake for 18–20 minutes, or until the fish flakes easily when tested with a fork.

5. Meanwhile, in a medium bowl, stir together the salsa ingredients.

6. Spoon the salsa on top of or alongside the fish.

Exchanges / Choices
1/2 Fruit, 4 Lean Meat

Calories	200	**Sodium**	220 mg
Calories from Fat	45	**Potassium**	790 mg
Total Fat	5 g	**Total Carbohydrate**	11 g
Saturated Fat	1 g	Dietary Fiber	2 g
Trans Fat	0 g	Sugars	6 g
Polyunsaturated Fat	1.5 g	**Protein**	30 g
Monounsaturated Fat	2 g	**Phosphorus**	360 mg
Cholesterol	100 mg		

BROILED ORANGE ROUGHY PARMESAN

Serves 4 / Serving Size: 3 ounces fish

A seasoned Parmesan and sour cream topping—ready in minutes—adds richness to mild orange roughy. Serve this savory fish dish with Thyme-Tinged Squash (page 145) or on a bed of Italian Skillet Spinach (page 143).

Cooking spray

1/3 cup fat-free sour cream

2 tablespoons shredded or grated Parmesan cheese

1 1/2 teaspoons fresh lemon juice

1/2 teaspoon garlic powder

1/2 teaspoon dried basil, crumbled

1/4 teaspoon onion powder

1/8 teaspoon pepper

1/8 teaspoon salt

4 orange roughy or other mild white fish fillets (about 4 ounces each), rinsed and patted dry

Exchanges / Choices
3 Lean Meat

Calories	120	Sodium	200 mg
Calories from Fat	20	Potassium	230 mg
Total Fat	**2 g**	**Total Carbohydrate**	**4 g**
Saturated Fat	0.5 g	Dietary Fiber	0 g
Trans Fat	0 g	Sugars	0 g
Polyunsaturated Fat	0 g	**Protein**	**20 g**
Monounsaturated Fat	0.5 g	**Phosphorus**	**160 mg**
Cholesterol	**70 mg**		

1. Preheat the broiler. Lightly spray a baking sheet with cooking spray.

2. Meanwhile, in a small bowl, whisk together all the ingredients except the fish. Set aside.

3. Place the fish on the baking sheet. Broil 2–3 inches from the heat for 3 minutes on each side. Remove from the oven. Spread the sour cream mixture over the top and sides of the fish. Broil for 30 seconds–1 minute, or until the topping is browned and the fish flakes easily when tested with a fork.

SALMON BAKED WITH CUCUMBERS AND DILL

Serves 4 / Serving Size: 3 ounces fish and 1/2 cup vegetables

Cucumbers, red onion, dill, and lemon are traditional accompaniments for smoked salmon, but they're just as delectable when baked with fresh fillets. Serve this with brown rice, quinoa, or the whole grain of your choice.

Cooking spray

2 small cucumbers, peeled and ends trimmed

1/2 small red onion, finely chopped

4 salmon fillets (about 4 ounces each), rinsed and patted dry

2 tablespoons fresh lemon or lime juice

1/4 cup loosely packed chopped fresh dillweed

1/4 teaspoon salt

1/4 teaspoon pepper

Exchanges / Choices
1 Vegetable, 4 Lean Meat

Calories	200	**Sodium**	165 mg
Calories from Fat	60	**Potassium**	805 mg
Total Fat	**7 g**	**Total Carbohydrate**	**6 g**
Saturated Fat	1.5 g	Dietary Fiber	2 g
Trans Fat	0 g	Sugars	3 g
Polyunsaturated Fat	2.5 g	**Protein**	**26 g**
Monounsaturated Fat	2.5 g	**Phosphorus**	**340 mg**
Cholesterol	**50 mg**		

1. Preheat the oven to 400°F. Lightly spray an 11 × 7 × 2-inch baking dish with cooking spray.

2. Cut each cucumber in half lengthwise. Scoop out and discard the seeds. Slice the cucumbers into 1/4-inch-thick crescents. Arrange the cucumbers and onion around the edges of the baking dish.

3. Place the fish in the center of the dish. Sprinkle the lemon juice over the fish. Sprinkle the remaining ingredients over the fish, cucumbers, and onion.

4. Bake for 15–20 minutes, or until the fish is cooked to the desired doneness and the vegetables are tender-crisp.

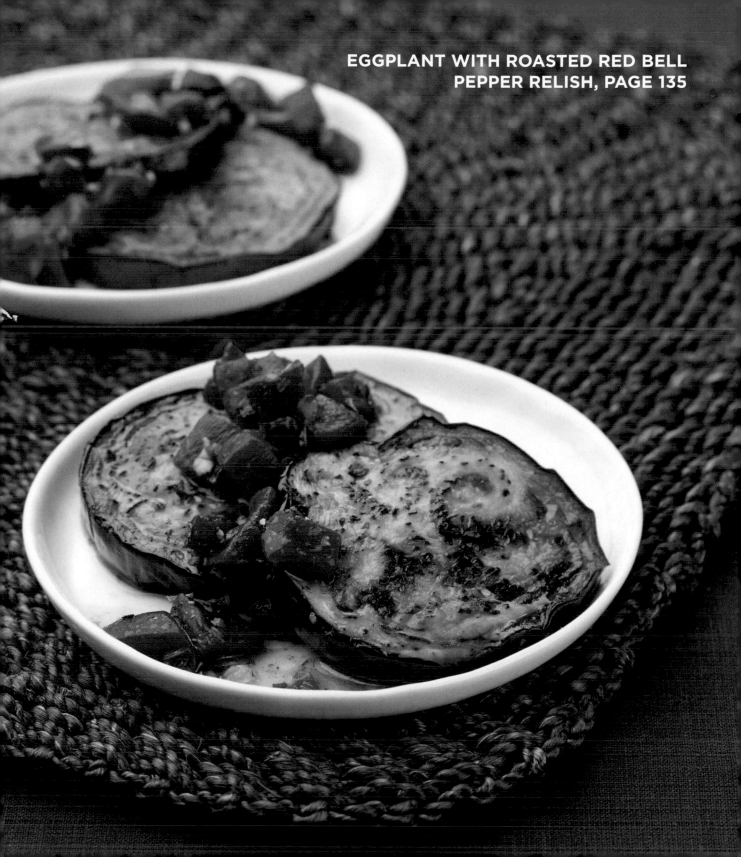

EGGPLANT WITH ROASTED RED BELL PEPPER RELISH, PAGE 135

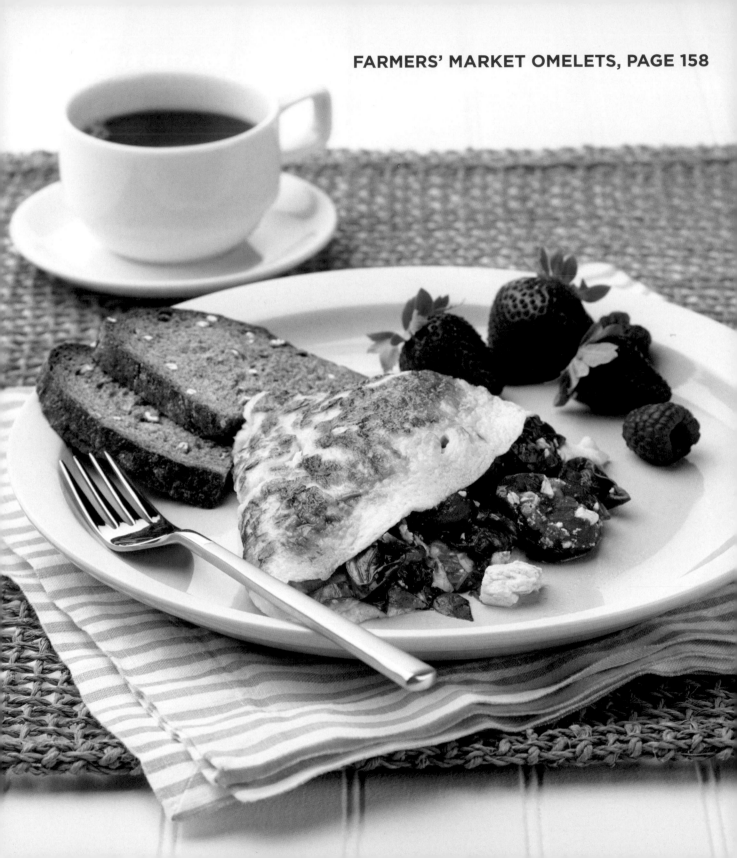

FARMERS' MARKET OMELETS, PAGE 158

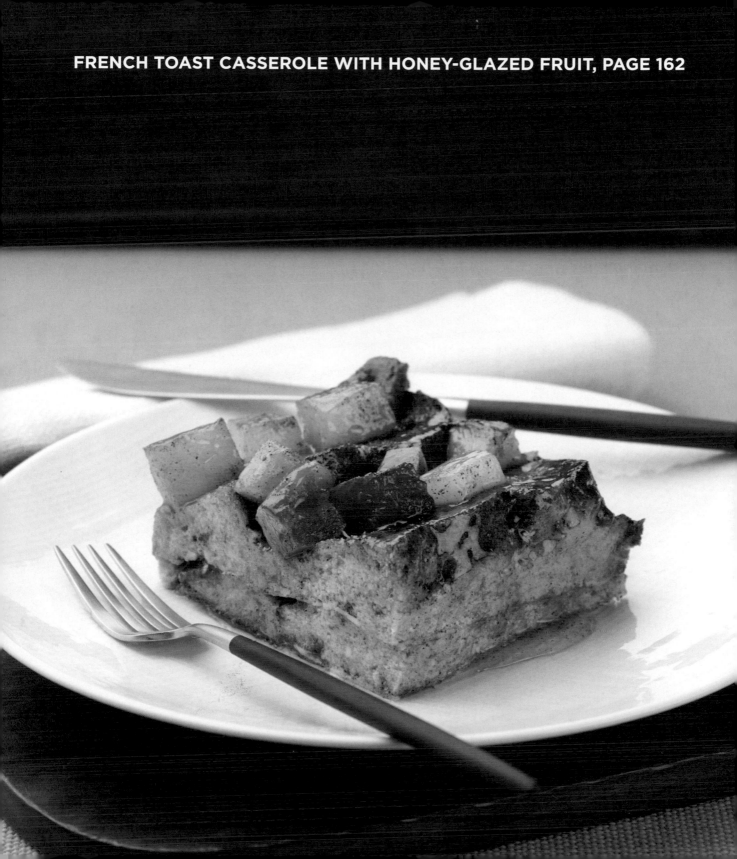

FRENCH TOAST CASSEROLE WITH HONEY-GLAZED FRUIT, PAGE 162

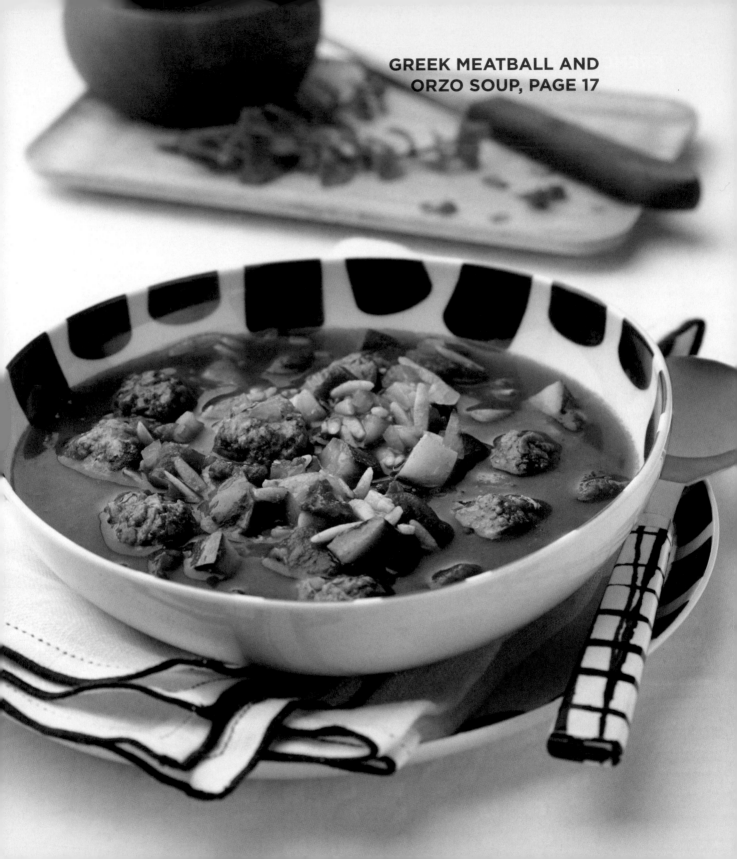

GREEK MEATBALL AND
ORZO SOUP, PAGE 17

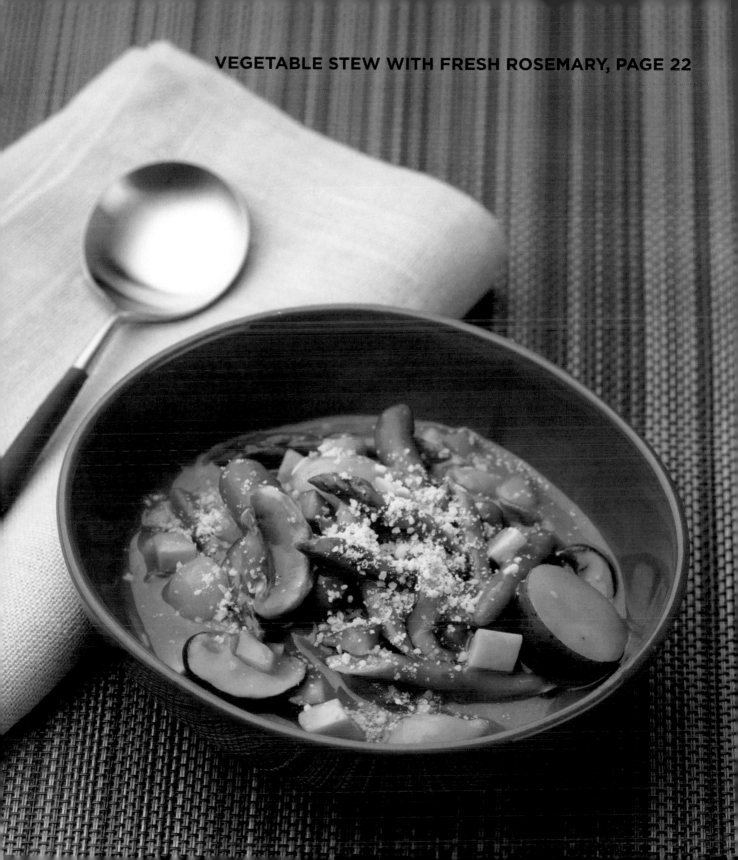

VEGETABLE STEW WITH FRESH ROSEMARY, PAGE 22

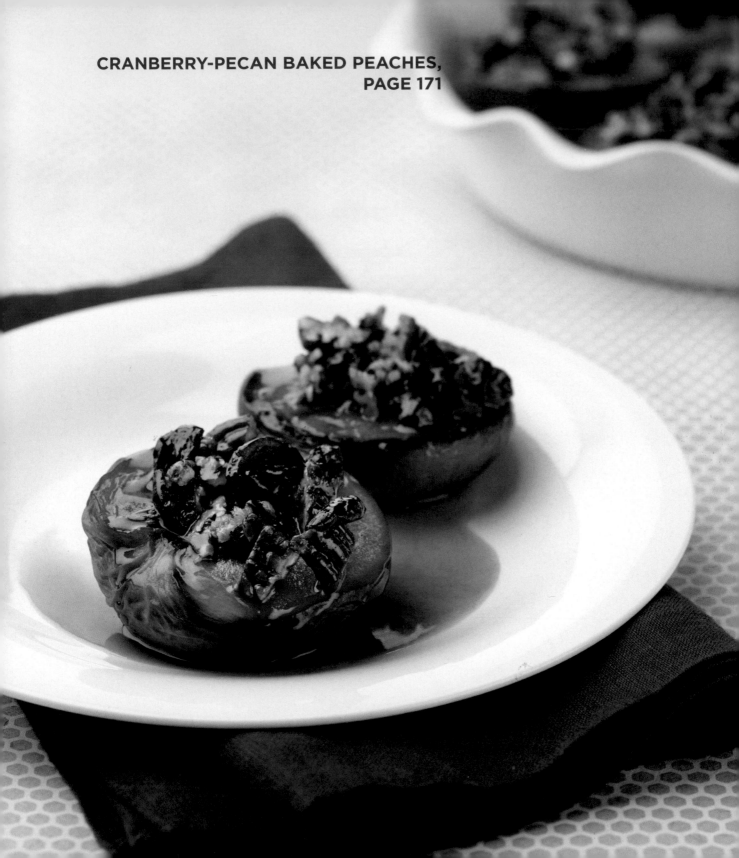

CRANBERRY-PECAN BAKED PEACHES,
PAGE 171

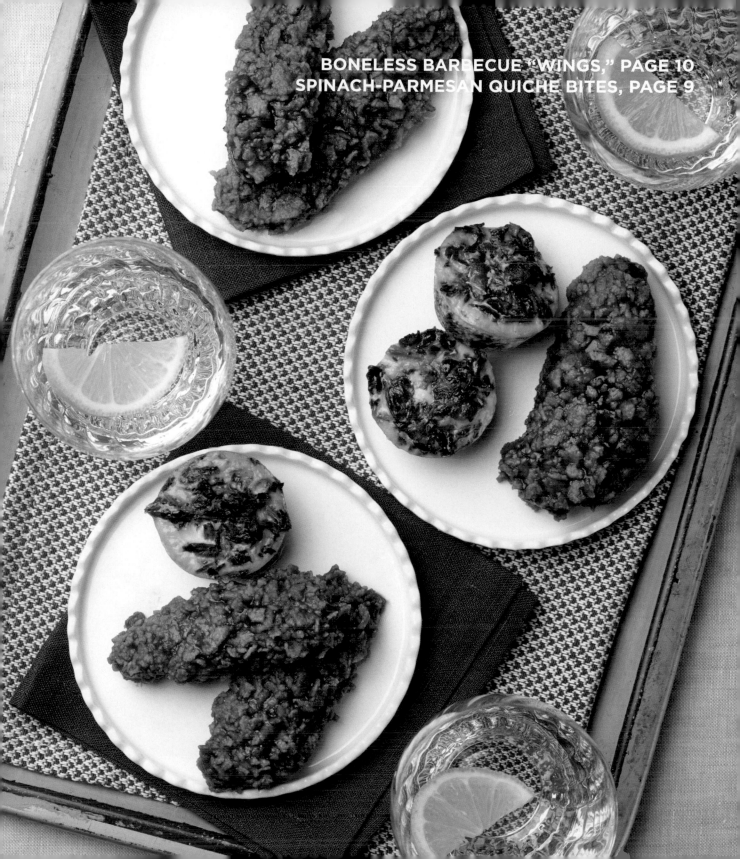

BONELESS BARBECUE "WINGS," PAGE 10
SPINACH-PARMESAN QUICHE BITES, PAGE 9

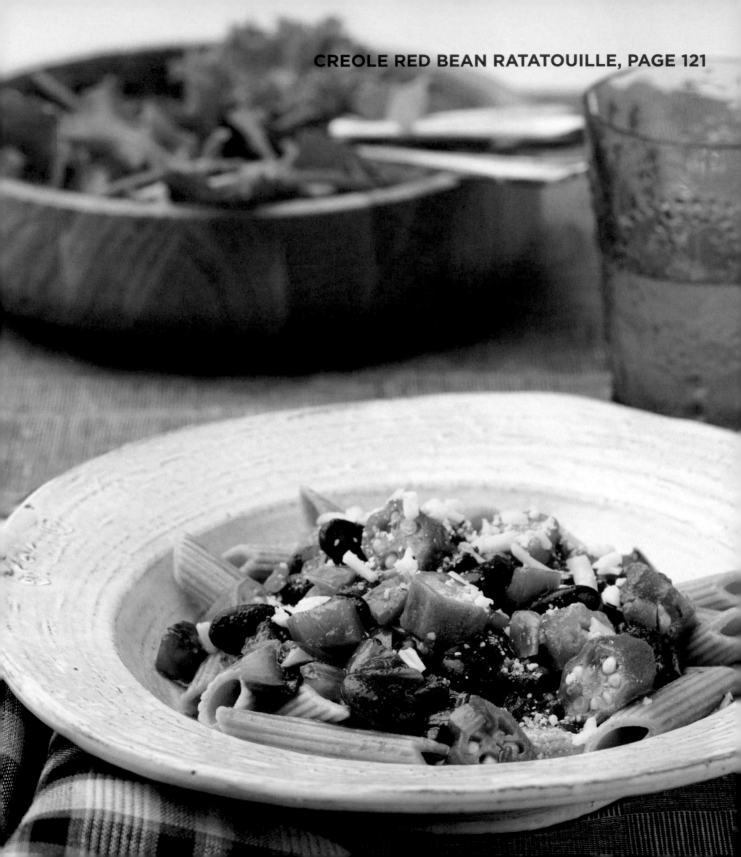

CREOLE RED BEAN RATATOUILLE, PAGE 121

SALMON WITH MANGO AND PEACH SALSA

Serves 4 / Serving Size: 3 ounces fish and 2 tablespoons salsa

Packed with the natural sweetness of mango and peaches, the salsa in this dish gets its kick from jalapeño and cumin. It's the perfect foil for the richness of salmon.

Cooking spray

Salsa

1 cup chopped peeled peaches or 1 (8-ounce) can peaches packed in water, drained and chopped

1 medium mango, chopped

1/4 cup chopped fresh cilantro

3 tablespoons chopped red onion

1 small fresh jalapeño, seeds and ribs discarded, chopped

1 teaspoon grated lime zest

2 tablespoons fresh lime juice

1/4 teaspoon ground cumin

1/4 teaspoon salt

1/4 teaspoon pepper (white preferred)

4 salmon fillets with skin (about 5 ounces each), rinsed and patted dry

1. Lightly spray the grill rack with cooking spray. Preheat the grill on medium high. Or lightly spray a grill pan with cooking spray and heat over medium-high heat.

2. In a medium bowl, stir together the salsa ingredients. Set aside.

3. Sprinkle the salt and pepper over the fish. Using your fingertips, gently press the seasonings so they adhere to the fish.

4. Grill the fish with the skin side up for 4 minutes, or until browned. Using a spatula, turn over. Grill for 3–4 minutes, or until the desired doneness.

5. Transfer the fish with the skin side down to plates. Spoon the salsa on top of or alongside the fish.

Exchanges / Choices			
1 Fruit, 4 Lean Meat			
Calories	260	Sodium	170 mg
Calories from Fat	80	Potassium	790 mg
Total Fat	9 g	Total Carbohydrate	13 g
Saturated Fat	2 g	Dietary Fiber	2 g
Trans Fat	0 g	Sugars	11 g
Polyunsaturated Fat	3 g	Protein	32 g
Monounsaturated Fat	3 g	Phosphorus	390 mg
Cholesterol	60 mg		

SALMON TACOS

Soft tortillas envelop a filling of tender grilled salmon, crunchy Mexican-spiced slaw, juicy tomato, and cool sour cream.

Cooking spray

1/4 cup fat-free plain yogurt

1 teaspoon grated lime zest

2 teaspoons fresh lime juice

1/4 teaspoon chili powder

1 1/2 cups shredded green cabbage or green-leaf lettuce

1/4 medium red or green bell pepper, chopped

2 tablespoons finely chopped red onion

1 1/2 teaspoons grated radish

1 teaspoon minced fresh jalapeño, seeds and ribs discarded

12 ounces salmon or cod fillets, rinsed, patted dry, and cut into 4 pieces

4 (6-inch) whole-grain tortillas (lowest sodium available)

1/2 cup chopped tomato

2 tablespoons fat-free sour cream

2 teaspoons chopped fresh cilantro

1. Lightly spray a grill pan with cooking spray and heat over medium-high heat. Or lightly spray the grill rack with cooking spray. Preheat the grill on medium high.

2. Meanwhile, in a small bowl, whisk together the yogurt, lime zest, and chili powder.

3. In a medium bowl, stir together the cabbage, bell pepper, onion, radish, and jalapeño. Add the yogurt mixture, tossing gently to coat. Set aside.

4. Grill the fish for 4 minutes on each side, or until the desired doneness. Transfer to a plate. Cover to keep warm.

5. Warm the tortillas using the package directions.

6. Transfer the tortillas to plates. Spoon the slaw down the center of each tortilla. Break the fish into chunks. Put the fish on the slaw. Sprinkle with the tomato.

7. In a small bowl, stir together the sour cream, lime juice, and cilantro. Spoon over the taco filling. Fold the sides of the tortillas over the filling.

Exchanges / Choices

1 1/2 Starch, 3 Lean Meat

Calories	240	**Sodium**	160 mg
Calories from Fat	50	**Potassium**	580 mg
Total Fat	6 g	**Total Carbohydrate**	25 g
Saturated Fat	1 g	Dietary Fiber	1 g
Trans Fat	0 g	Sugars	4 g
Polyunsaturated Fat	2 g	**Protein**	22 g
Monounsaturated Fat	2 g	**Phosphorus**	300 mg
Cholesterol	40 mg		

SALMON CROQUETTES WITH YOGURT-HORSERADISH SAUCE

Serves 6 / Serving Size: 1 croquette and 2 tablespoons sauce

A zippy horseradish-infused yogurt sauce enlivens the down-home flavor of crisp croquettes. They're great hot, at room temperature, or chilled. A green salad, such as Salad Greens with Mixed-Herb Vinaigrette (page 25), is all you need to turn these into a light but satisfying meal.

Sauce

1/2 cup fat-free plain yogurt

2 tablespoons chopped fresh Italian (flat-leaf) parsley

1 tablespoon bottled white horseradish, drained

1 tablespoon grated onion

Croquettes

1 (14.5-ounce) can boneless, skinless red or pink salmon, drained and flaked

1/2 cup chopped red bell pepper

1/3 cup crushed whole-grain crispbread (lowest sodium available)

1/4 cup chopped red onion

1 large egg

1 1/2 teaspoons chopped fresh dillweed or 1/2 teaspoon dried dillweed, crumbled

1/4 teaspoon pepper

2 teaspoons canola or corn oil

1. In a small bowl, stir together the sauce ingredients. Cover and refrigerate.

2. In a medium bowl, stir together the croquette ingredients except the oil. Shape into 6 patties, each about 3 inches in diameter.

3. In a large skillet, heat the oil over medium-high heat, swirling to coat the bottom. Cook the croquettes for 2–3 minutes on each side, or until golden brown.

4. Transfer the croquettes to plates. Spoon the sauce alongside or on top of the croquettes.

Cook's Tip on Making Crispbread Crumbs: It's about as easy to crush an entire box of crispbread as to do just the amount a recipe calls for. Process several pieces in a food processor or blender until you have fine crumbs. Repeat the procedure with the remaining pieces. Use what you need, and freeze the rest in an airtight freezer bag or a freezer-proof container with a tight-fitting lid.

Exchanges / Choices
1 Carbohydrate, 3 Lean Meat

Calories	210	**Sodium**	360 mg
Calories from Fat	60	**Potassium**	410 mg
Total Fat	7 g	**Total Carbohydrate**	15 g
Saturated Fat	1 g	Dietary Fiber	3 g
Trans Fat	0 g	Sugars	3 g
Polyunsaturated Fat	2 g	**Protein**	22 g
Monounsaturated Fat	3 g	**Phosphorus**	270 mg
Cholesterol	80 mg		

TILAPIA WITH DILL AND PAPRIKA

Serves 4 / Serving Size: 3 ounces fish

Sometimes simple is best, as in this lightly seasoned fish dish. Tilapia gets a classic treatment when it's baked with a touch of dill and a sprinkle of colorful paprika. A squeeze of lemon at serving time adds a bit of brightness. Because the flavors are so mild, this entrée pairs well with almost any side dish, such as Tarragon Tomatoes (page 148) or Red Potatoes Parmesan (page 140).

Olive oil cooking spray

4 tilapia or other thin, mild fish fillets (about 4 ounces each), rinsed and patted dry

1 teaspoon dried dillweed, crumbled

3/4 teaspoon paprika

1/4 teaspoon salt

1/4 teaspoon pepper

2 medium lemons, each cut into 4 wedges

Exchanges / Choices

3 Lean Meat

Calories	120	**Sodium**	160 mg
Calories from Fat	20	**Potassium**	370 mg
Total Fat	2 g	**Total Carbohydrate**	1 g
Saturated Fat	1 g	Dietary Fiber	0 g
Trans Fat	0 g	Sugars	0 g
Polyunsaturated Fat	0.5 g	**Protein**	24 g
Monounsaturated Fat	0.5 g	**Phosphorus**	200 mg
Cholesterol	60 mg		

1. Preheat the oven to 350°F. Lightly spray a baking sheet with cooking spray. Place the fish on the baking sheet.

2. In a small bowl, stir together the dillweed, paprika, salt, and pepper. Sprinkle over the fish. Lightly spray the fish with cooking spray.

3. Bake for 10–12 minutes, or until the fish flakes easily when tested with a fork.

4. Serve with the lemon wedges.

LEMONY TILAPIA AND ASPARAGUS GRILL

Serves 4 / Serving Size: 3 ounces fish and 6 asparagus spears

Dinner is incredibly quick and easy when you grill tilapia and asparagus side by side. A combination of chili powder and lemon pepper enhances the mild fish, and a simple vinaigrette seasons the spears. *(See photo insert.)*

Cooking spray

1 tablespoon olive oil

1 tablespoon red wine vinegar

1 1/2 teaspoons salt-free lemon pepper, divided use

1 1/4 teaspoons garlic powder, divided use

1 pound asparagus spears (about 24), trimmed

1 1/2 tablespoons chili powder

1/8 teaspoon cayenne

1/8 teaspoon salt

4 tilapia fillets (about 4 ounces each), rinsed and patted dry

1 medium lemon, cut into 4 wedges

1. Lightly spray the grill rack with cooking spray. Preheat the grill on medium high.

2. Meanwhile, in a small bowl, whisk together the oil, vinegar, 1/2 teaspoon lemon pepper, and 1/2 teaspoon garlic powder. Pour into a large shallow casserole dish. Add the asparagus, turning several times to coat.

3. In a small bowl, stir together the chili powder, cayenne, salt, and the remaining 1 teaspoon lemon pepper and 3/4 teaspoon garlic powder. Sprinkle over both sides of the fish. Using your fingertips, gently press the mixture so it adheres to the fish. Lightly spray both sides of the fish with cooking spray.

4. Drain the asparagus, discarding the marinade.

5. Place the fish and asparagus lengthwise so they are perpendicular to the grates of the grill. (For the fish, you can also use a grill basket lightly sprayed with cooking spray.) Grill the fish for 3 minutes on each side, or until it flakes easily when tested with a fork. Grill the asparagus for 4–5 minutes, or until tender, turning frequently. Transfer both to a platter. Serve with the lemon wedges.

Exchanges / Choices

2 Vegetable, 3 Lean Meat

Calories	180	Sodium	210 mg
Calories from Fat	50	Potassium	680 mg
Total Fat	**6 g**	**Total Carbohydrate**	**9 g**
Saturated Fat	1 g	Dietary Fiber	5 g
Trans Fat	0 g	Sugars	3 g
Polyunsaturated Fat	1 g	**Protein**	**26 g**
Monounsaturated Fat	3.5 g	**Phosphorus**	**270 mg**
Cholesterol	**60 mg**		

GRILLED TROUT AMANDINE WITH GINGER AND ORANGE

Serves 4 / Serving Size: 3 ounces fish

Ginger, thyme, and orange infuse trout fillets with flavor, while a topping of dry-roasted almonds adds texture. Steamed red potatoes and asparagus or sugar snap peas make fine partners.

Cooking spray

1 teaspoon grated orange zest

2 tablespoons fresh orange juice

2 teaspoons canola or corn oil

1 1/2 teaspoons minced peeled gingerroot or 1/2 teaspoon ground ginger

1 1/2 teaspoons chopped fresh thyme or 1/2 teaspoon dried thyme, crumbled

1/4 teaspoon pepper

1/8 teaspoon salt

4 rainbow trout fillets with skin (about 5 ounces each), rinsed and patted dry

3 tablespoons slivered almonds, dry-roasted

1. Lightly spray a stovetop grill with cooking spray and heat over medium-high heat. Or lightly spray the grill rack with cooking spray. Preheat the grill on medium high.

2. In a small bowl, whisk together the orange zest, orange juice, oil, gingerroot, thyme, pepper, and salt. Brush the mixture over the flesh side of the fish.

3. Grill the fish with the flesh side down for 3 minutes. Turn over. Grill for 1–3 minutes, or until the fish flakes easily when tested with a fork.

4. Discard the skin. Just before serving, sprinkle with the almonds.

Cook's Tip on Trout: Trout is a freshwater fish related to salmon. Rainbow and steelhead are two popular varieties. Trout is sold both fresh and frozen year-round. When defrosting frozen trout or other seafood, follow the package directions carefully. Rinse the fish and dry it thoroughly with several layers of paper towels. The fish will have retained a lot of water from being frozen and should be thoroughly dry before you coat or cook it.

Exchanges / Choices
4 Lean Meat, 1 Fat

Calories	230	**Sodium**	95 mg
Calories from Fat	90	**Potassium**	740 mg
Total Fat	**10 g**	**Total Carbohydrate**	**2 g**
Saturated Fat	1.5 g	Dietary Fiber	1 g
Trans Fat	0 g	Sugars	1 g
Polyunsaturated Fat	3 g	**Protein**	**30 g**
Monounsaturated Fat	5 g	**Phosphorus**	410 mg
Cholesterol	**80 mg**		

TUNA KEBABS

Serves 6 / Serving Size: 1 kebab

When you're looking to cook out, try fresh tuna flavored with an Asian-style marinade and skewered with bell peppers, tender squash, crunchy red onion, and succulent tomatoes and pineapple. *(See photo insert.)*

Marinade

1/4 cup chopped green onions

3 tablespoons 100% pineapple juice

1 1/2 tablespoons soy sauce (lowest sodium available)

1 tablespoon red wine vinegar or rice vinegar

1 tablespoon water

1 tablespoon honey

1 medium garlic clove, minced

1/2 teaspoon ground ginger

1/4 teaspoon pepper

1 pound tuna steaks, rinsed, patted dry, and cut into 12 cubes

Cooking spray

1 small red or green bell pepper, cut into 12 squares

1 small yellow summer squash or zucchini, cut into 12 slices

1 small red onion, cut into 12 wedges

12 (1 1/2-inch) cubes pineapple

12 grape or cherry tomatoes

1. In a large glass baking dish, stir together the marinade ingredients. Remove and set aside 2 tablespoons of the marinade.

2. Add the fish to the marinade remaining in the dish, turning to coat. Cover and refrigerate for 15 minutes–1 hour, turning occasionally.

3. Drain the fish, discarding the marinade. Pat the fish dry with paper towels.

4. Lightly spray the grill rack with cooking spray. Preheat the grill on medium high. Or lightly spray a large indoor grill pan with cooking spray. Heat over medium-high heat.

5. Meanwhile, soak six 12-inch wooden skewers for at least 10 minutes in cold water to keep them from charring, or use metal skewers. Lightly spray the skewers with cooking spray. For each kebab, thread each skewer with 2 tuna cubes, 2 bell pepper squares, 2 slices of squash, 2 onion wedges, 2 pineapple cubes, and 2 tomatoes. Baste with the reserved marinade.

6. Grill the kebabs for 4 minutes. Turn over. Grill for 3–5 minutes, or until the fish is cooked to the desired doneness.

Exchanges / Choices
2 Vegetable, 2 Lean Meat

Calories	140	**Sodium**	190 mg
Calories from Fat	10	**Potassium**	630 mg
Total Fat	1 g	**Total Carbohydrate**	14 g
Saturated Fat	0 g	Dietary Fiber	2 g
Trans Fat	0 g	Sugars	10 g
Polyunsaturated Fat	0 g	**Protein**	20 g
Monounsaturated Fat	0 g	**Phosphorus**	250 mg
Cholesterol	30 mg		

TUNA-MACARONI CASSEROLE

Serves 4 / Serving Size: 1 1/2 cups

Can the canned soup. A classic one-dish meal gets a modern-day makeover with whole-grain pasta, chickpeas, fresh vegetables, and a zesty tomato-based sauce.

1 cup dried whole-grain elbow macaroni or small shell pasta

Cooking spray

2 teaspoons olive oil

1 medium onion, chopped

1 medium rib of celery, chopped

1 small red or green bell pepper, chopped

2 medium garlic cloves, minced

1 (14.5-ounce) can no-salt-added diced tomatoes, undrained

2 tablespoons chopped fresh basil or 2 teaspoons dried basil, crumbled

2 tablespoons no-salt-added tomato paste

1 tablespoon red wine vinegar

1/4 teaspoon salt

1/8 teaspoon cayenne

2 (4.5-ounce) cans very low sodium albacore tuna, packed in water, drained and flaked

1 cup no-salt-added canned chickpeas, rinsed and drained

3 tablespoons shredded or grated Parmesan cheese

1. Prepare the pasta using the package directions, omitting the salt. Drain well in a colander. Transfer to a large bowl.

2. Preheat the oven to 375°F. Lightly spray an 11 x 7 x 2-inch baking dish with cooking spray.

3. In a Dutch oven, heat the oil over medium-high heat, swirling to coat the bottom. Cook the onion, celery, bell pepper, and garlic for 3 minutes, or until the onion is soft, stirring frequently.

4. Stir in the tomatoes with liquid, basil, tomato paste, vinegar, salt, and cayenne. Cook for 3 minutes, stirring frequently. Stir the tomato mixture into the pasta.

5. Stir the tuna and chickpeas into the pasta mixture. Spoon into the baking dish.

6. Bake for 10 minutes. Stir. Bake for 10–15 minutes, or until the casserole is very hot and most of the liquid is absorbed. Sprinkle with the Parmesan. Bake for 5 minutes, or until the Parmesan has melted and is lightly golden.

Exchanges / Choices
2 Starch, 2 Vegetable, 3 Lean Meat

Calories	330	**Sodium**	330 mg
Calories from Fat	60	**Potassium**	860 mg
Total Fat	**7 g**	**Total Carbohydrate**	**44 g**
Saturated Fat	1.5 g	Dietary Fiber	8 g
Trans Fat	0 g	Sugars	10 g
Polyunsaturated Fat	1.5 g	**Protein**	**26 g**
Monounsaturated Fat	3 g	**Phosphorus**	**300 mg**
Cholesterol	**30 mg**		

SKILLET-FRIED OYSTERS WITH DIJON SOUR CREAM

Serves 4 / Serving Size: 8 oysters and 2 tablespoons sauce

Sweet, toothsome oysters are bathed in a spicy, crunchy coating and served with a zesty sour cream sauce. Try them with another southern-style favorite, Down-Home Greens (page 138), or baked sweet potato fries.

1/3 cup fat-free sour cream

2 teaspoons Dijon mustard (lowest sodium available)

1 1/2 teaspoons olive oil (extra virgin preferred)

1/4 teaspoon salt

1/4 teaspoon pepper

1/2 cup yellow cornmeal

1 teaspoon paprika

1 teaspoon salt-free Creole or Cajun seasoning blend (see Cook's Tip on Creole or Cajun Seasoning Blend, page 38)

32 shucked raw medium oysters, drained (about 1 pound)

2 tablespoons canola or corn oil

Exchanges / Choices

1 1/2 Carbohydrate, 2 Lean Meat, 1 Fat

Calories	240	Sodium	320 mg
Calories from Fat	110	Potassium	275 mg
Total Fat	**12 g**	**Total Carbohydrate**	**21 g**
Saturated Fat	1.5 g	Dietary Fiber	1 g
Trans Fat	0 g	Sugars	0 g
Polyunsaturated Fat	3.5 g	**Protein**	**13 g**
Monounsaturated Fat	6 g	**Phosphorus**	**240 mg**
Cholesterol	**60 mg**		

1. In a small bowl, whisk together the sour cream, mustard, olive oil, salt, and pepper. Set aside.

2. In a shallow dish or pie pan, stir together the cornmeal, paprika, and seasoning blend. Dip the oysters in the cornmeal mixture, turning to coat and gently shaking off the excess. Transfer to a large plate.

3. In a large nonstick skillet, heat the canola oil over medium-high heat, swirling to coat the bottom. Cook the oysters for 4 minutes, turning frequently.

4. Serve with the sour cream mixture.

PARSLEY PESTO SHRIMP

Serves 4 / Serving Size: 1/2 cup shrimp mixture and 1/2 cup rice

Shrimp is tossed in a mixture of lemon, garlic, parsley, and olive oil, and then served over rice to catch all the savory sauce. A smidge of red pepper adds just the right amount of heat. Add Italian Skillet Spinach (page 143) for a dinner that's ready in a flash.

1/2 cup uncooked instant brown rice

1/4 cup minced fresh parsley

1 teaspoon grated lemon zest

3 tablespoons fresh lemon juice

2 tablespoons olive oil

1 medium garlic clove, minced

1/4 teaspoon crushed red pepper flakes

1/8 teaspoon salt

Cooking spray

12 ounces raw medium shrimp, peeled, rinsed, and patted dry

1 medium lemon, cut into 4 wedges

Exchanges / Choices
1 1/2 Starch, 2 Lean Meat 1/2 Fat

Calories	220	Sodium	490 mg
Calories from Fat	80	Potassium	235 mg
Total Fat	**9 g**	**Total Carbohydrate**	**23 g**
Saturated Fat	1.5 g	Dietary Fiber	2 g
Trans Fat	0 g	Sugars	1 g
Polyunsaturated Fat	1.5 g	**Protein**	**14 g**
Monounsaturated Fat	6 g	**Phosphorus**	**280 mg**
Cholesterol	**110 mg**		

1. Prepare the rice using the package directions, omitting the salt and margarine.

2. Meanwhile, in a small bowl, stir together the parsley, lemon zest, lemon juice, oil, garlic, red pepper flakes, and salt.

3. When the rice is almost ready, lightly spray a large skillet with cooking spray. Cook the shrimp over medium heat for 4 minutes, or until pink on the outside, stirring frequently. Remove from the heat. Gently stir in the parsley mixture.

4. Spoon the rice onto plates. Spoon the shrimp mixture over the rice. Serve with the lemon wedges.

DEEP-SOUTH SHRIMP GUMBO

Serves 6 / Serving Size: 1 cup gumbo and 1/2 cup rice

Browning the flour helps to deepen the flavor of this classic Louisiana stew, filled with tender vegetables and shrimp. The combination of bell pepper, onion, and celery is a staple in Cajun and Creole cooking.

1/4 cup all-purpose flour

2 teaspoons canola or corn oil

1 large onion, chopped

1 medium green bell pepper, chopped

1 1/2 medium ribs of celery, chopped

1 (14.5-ounce) can no-salt-added stewed tomatoes, undrained

10 ounces frozen cut okra

1 3/4 cups fat-free, low-sodium chicken broth, divided use

2 medium dried bay leaves

1 teaspoon dried thyme, crumbled

1/4 teaspoon pepper

12 ounces raw medium shrimp, peeled, rinsed, and patted dry

1/2 teaspoon red hot-pepper sauce, or to taste

1 cup uncooked brown rice

1. Heat a Dutch oven over medium-high heat. Cook the flour for 2 minutes, or until golden, stirring constantly with a flat spatula to prevent scorching. Transfer the flour to a small bowl.

2. In the same pot, still over medium-high heat, heat the oil, swirling to coat the bottom. Cook the onion, bell pepper, and celery for 2 minutes, or until the onion is tender, stirring frequently.

3. Stir in the tomatoes with liquid, okra, 1 1/4 cups broth, bay leaves, thyme, and pepper.

4. Stir the remaining 1/2 cup broth into the flour to make a thick paste. Add the flour mixture to the tomato mixture, stirring until well blended. Bring to a boil. Reduce the heat and simmer, covered, for 30 minutes, or until the okra is very tender.

5. Stir in the shrimp. Simmer for 5 minutes, or until the shrimp are pink on the outside. Remove from the heat. Stir in the hot-pepper sauce. Let stand, covered, for 30 minutes. Discard the bay leaves.

6. Meanwhile, prepare the rice using the package directions, omitting the salt and margarine.

7. Just before serving, reheat the gumbo over low heat if necessary. Spoon the rice into bowls. Ladle the gumbo over the rice.

Exchanges / Choices
2 Starch, 3 Vegetable, 1 Lean Meat

Calories	260	Sodium	400 mg
Calories from Fat	35	Potassium	590 mg
Total Fat	**4 g**	**Total Carbohydrate**	**43 g**
Saturated Fat	0.5 g	Dietary Fiber	4 g
Trans Fat	0 g	Sugars	8 g
Polyunsaturated Fat	1 g	**Protein**	**14 g**
Monounsaturated Fat	1.5 g	**Phosphorus**	**300 mg**
Cholesterol	**70 mg**		

| *Poultry* |

ROAST CHICKEN BREASTS WITH VEGETABLE MEDLEY

Serves 4 / Serving Size: 3 ounces chicken and 1 cup vegetables

Chicken and vegetables are roasted with a savory combination of orange juice, garlic, and fresh thyme. Everything comes out of the oven at about the same time, making it easy to put a complete meal on the table.

Cooking spray

3 tablespoons fresh orange juice, divided use

2 teaspoons olive oil

3 medium garlic cloves, minced, divided use

1 tablespoon plus 1 1/2 teaspoons minced fresh thyme, divided use

1/2 teaspoon pepper, divided use

1/4 teaspoon salt, divided use

1 medium leek (white part only), halved lengthwise, then cut crosswise into 1/2-inch pieces

1 medium sweet potato, peeled, halved lengthwise, then cut crosswise into 1/2-inch pieces

1 medium white potato, halved lengthwise, then cut crosswise into 1/2-inch pieces

1 medium red onion, cut into 12 wedges

1 cup baby carrots or 2 medium carrots, sliced

6 medium asparagus spears, trimmed and halved crosswise

4 chicken breast halves with bone and skin (about 6 ounces each), all visible fat discarded

1. Preheat the oven to 400°F. Lightly spray a metal baking pan with cooking spray. Place a rack in a roasting pan or separate metal baking pan. Lightly spray the rack with cooking spray.

2. In a large glass baking dish, stir together 2 tablespoons orange juice, the oil, 2 garlic cloves, 1 tablespoon thyme, 1/4 teaspoon pepper, and 1/8 teaspoon salt. Remove and set aside 2 teaspoons of the orange juice mixture.

3. Add the leek, both potatoes, onion, and carrots to the marinade in the baking dish, turning to coat.

4. Drain the vegetables, discarding the marinade. Arrange the vegetables in a single layer in the baking pan. Roast for 15 minutes.

5. Brush the asparagus with the reserved marinade. Set aside.

6. In a small bowl, stir together the remaining 1 tablespoon orange juice, 1 garlic clove, 1 1/2 teaspoons thyme, 1/4 teaspoon pepper, and 1/8 teaspoon salt. Put the chicken on a cutting board or flat work surface. Carefully loosen the skin from the chicken breasts by gently inserting your fingers between the skin and the meat, making a pocket for the orange juice mixture. Don't break the skin. Discard any fat beneath the skin. Still working carefully, spread the orange juice mixture under the loosened skin as well as possible. Transfer the chicken to the rack in the pan.

7. When the vegetables have roasted for 15 minutes, put the chicken in the oven. If the two pans don't fit on the same oven rack, use two racks, with the chicken on the upper rack. Roast for 25 minutes.

8. Add the asparagus to the pan with the vegetables, moving some of the other vegetables toward the sides of the pan so you can arrange the asparagus in a single layer. Roast the chicken and the vegetables for 10–12 minutes, or until the chicken is no longer pink in the center and all the vegetables are tender.

9. Just before serving, remove and discard the skin from the chicken.

Exchanges / Choices

1 1/2 Starch, 1 Vegetable, 4 Lean Meat

Calories	310	Sodium	310 mg
Calories from Fat	60	Potassium	1150 mg
Total Fat	**7 g**	**Total Carbohydrate**	**30 g**
Saturated Fat	1.5 g	Dietary Fiber	4 g
Trans Fat	0 g	Sugars	7 g
Polyunsaturated Fat	1 g	**Protein**	**34 g**
Monounsaturated Fat	3 g	**Phosphorus**	**390 mg**
Cholesterol	**90 mg**		

BAKED PARMESAN CHICKEN

Serves 4 / Serving Size: 3 ounces chicken

The crisp coating on this chicken is livened up with Parmesan, parsley, and oregano before it's baked to golden perfection. Whole-grain pasta and a salad of mixed greens and cherry tomatoes would complete the meal deliciously and nutritiously.

Cooking spray

1 large egg

1 tablespoon water

2 teaspoons olive oil

1/3 cup finely crushed whole-grain crispbread (lowest sodium available)

1/3 cup shredded or grated Parmesan cheese

2 tablespoons minced fresh parsley

1/2 teaspoon ground oregano

1/4 teaspoon pepper

4 boneless, skinless chicken breast halves (about 4 ounces each) or 1 pound boneless, skinless turkey breast, all visible fat discarded, flattened to 1/4-inch thickness

1. Preheat the oven to 400°F. Lightly spray a 13 × 9 × 2-inch baking dish with cooking spray.

2. In a shallow dish, whisk together the egg, water, and oil. In a separate shallow dish or pie pan, stir together the remaining ingredients except the chicken. Set the dishes and baking dish in a row, assembly-line fashion. Dip the chicken in the egg mixture, then in the crumb mixture, turning to coat at each step and gently shaking off any excess. Using your fingertips, gently press the coating mixture so it adheres to the chicken. Arrange the chicken in a single layer in the baking dish. Lightly spray the chicken with cooking spray.

3. Bake for 15–18 minutes, or until the chicken is no longer pink in the center and the top coating is golden brown.

Exchanges / Choices
1 Starch, 4 Lean Meat

Calories	**280**		**Sodium**	**340 mg**
Calories from Fat	80		**Potassium**	**530 mg**
Total Fat	**9 g**		**Total Carbohydrate**	**18 g**
Saturated Fat	2.5 g		Dietary Fiber	4 g
Trans Fat	0 g		Sugars	0 g
Polyunsaturated Fat	1 g		**Protein**	**30 g**
Monounsaturated Fat	4 g		**Phosphorus**	**370 mg**
Cholesterol	**125 mg**			

CHEESE-FILLED OVEN-FRIED CHICKEN

Serves 4 / Serving Size: 1 chicken roll

Crumb-topped chicken breasts hide a delicious secret—they're wrapped around gooey melted mozzarella cheese. Try them with Mediterranean Zucchini (page 149), which bakes at the same temperature and for the same amount of time.

Cooking spray

2 slices whole-grain bread (lowest sodium available), torn into small pieces

1 1/2 teaspoons dried basil, crumbled, divided use

3/4 teaspoon dried oregano, crumbled, divided use

1/4 teaspoon paprika

4 boneless, skinless chicken breast halves (about 4 ounces each), all visible fat discarded, flattened to 1/4-inch thickness

1 medium lemon, halved, divided use

1/4 cup chopped fresh parsley, divided use

4 low-fat mozzarella cheese sticks (string cheese)

1/8 teaspoon salt

1. Preheat the oven to 400°F. Lightly spray a baking sheet with cooking spray.

2. In a food processor or blender, process the bread, 1 teaspoon basil, 1/2 teaspoon oregano, and the paprika to the texture of coarse breadcrumbs.

3. Put the chicken on the baking sheet. Squeeze the juice of half a lemon over the chicken. Sprinkle with the remaining 1/2 teaspoon basil and 1/4 teaspoon oregano. Sprinkle with 2 tablespoons parsley. Place a cheese stick at one edge of each piece of chicken. Roll up jelly-roll style. Place with the seam side down on the baking sheet, leaving about 1/2 inch between the chicken rolls.

4. Squeeze the remaining lemon half over the rolls. Sprinkle with the bread crumb mixture. Sprinkle with the salt. Lightly spray the chicken with cooking spray.

5. Bake for 20 minutes, or until the chicken is no longer pink in the center. Just before serving, sprinkle with the remaining 2 tablespoons parsley.

Exchanges / Choices
1 Starch, 4 Lean Meat

Calories	210	**Sodium**	260 mg
Calories from Fat	50	**Potassium**	590 mg
Total Fat	5 g	**Total Carbohydrate**	12 g
Saturated Fat	1.5 g	Dietary Fiber	3 g
Trans Fat	0 g	Sugars	1 g
Polyunsaturated Fat	0.5 g	**Protein**	30 g
Monounsaturated Fat	1 g	**Phosphorus**	360 mg
Cholesterol	80 mg		

OVEN-FRIED SESAME-GINGER CHICKEN

Serves 4 / Serving Size: 3 ounces chicken

This chicken is crunchy, moist, and juicy, all at the same time, with a distinctly Asian flair from the soy sauce, gingerroot, and sesame. Serve it alongside brown rice and a green vegetable, such as Asian Broccoli with Pecans (page 134).

Cooking spray

1 large egg white

1 1/2 tablespoons soy or teriyaki sauce (lowest sodium available)

1 tablespoon cornstarch

1 tablespoon water

2 teaspoons canola or corn oil

1 teaspoon grated peeled gingerroot

1 medium garlic clove, crushed

1/4 teaspoon pepper

1/3 cup sesame seeds

4 boneless, skinless chicken breast halves (about 4 ounces each), all visible fat discarded

1. Preheat the oven to 400°F. Lightly spray an 11 × 7 × 2-inch baking dish with cooking spray.

2. In a shallow dish, whisk together the egg white, soy sauce, cornstarch, water, oil, gingerroot, garlic, and pepper. Put the sesame seeds in a separate shallow dish. Set the dishes and baking dish in a row, assembly-line fashion. Dip the chicken in the egg white mixture, then in the sesame seeds, turning to coat at each step and gently shaking off any excess. Arrange the chicken in a single layer in the baking dish.

3. Bake for 25–30 minutes, or until the chicken is no longer pink in the center and the top coating is crisp.

Cook's Tip: The texture of cornstarch is a bit finer than that of flour and gives the chicken a more delicate crust.

Exchanges / Choices
1/2 Starch, 4 Lean Meat, 1/2 Fat

Calories	240	**Sodium**	370 mg
Calories from Fat	100	**Potassium**	510 mg
Total Fat	11 g	**Total Carbohydrate**	6 g
Saturated Fat	1.5 g	Dietary Fiber	2 g
Trans Fat	0 g	Sugars	0 g
Polyunsaturated Fat	3.5 g	**Protein**	28 g
Monounsaturated Fat	4.5 g	**Phosphorus**	325 mg
Cholesterol	70 mg		

TEX-MEX CHICKEN FINGERS

Serves 4 / Serving Size: 3 ounces chicken

A favorite menu item at many restaurants, chicken fingers are easy to prepare healthfully at home. Serve them with some raw carrots, celery, and bell pepper strips, and a creamy dip, such as Triple-Duty Ranch Dip with Dill (page 4).

Cooking spray

1/3 cup low-fat buttermilk

1 teaspoon grated lime zest

1 tablespoon fresh lime juice

1/2 cup yellow cornmeal

2 tablespoons chopped fresh cilantro

1/2 teaspoon chili powder

1/2 teaspoon ground cumin

1/2 teaspoon dried oregano, crumbled

1/8 teaspoon cayenne

1 pound boneless, skinless chicken breasts or tenders, all visible fat discarded, cut into strips if breasts

1. Preheat the oven to 400°F. Lightly spray an 11 × 7 × 2-inch baking dish with cooking spray.

2. In a shallow dish, whisk together the buttermilk, lime zest, and lime juice. In a separate shallow dish, stir together the cornmeal, cilantro, chili powder, cumin, oregano, and cayenne. Set the dishes and baking dish in a row, assembly-line fashion. Dip the chicken in the buttermilk mixture, then in the cornmeal mixture, turning to coat at each step and gently shaking off any excess. Using your fingertips, gently press the coating mixture so it adheres to the chicken. Arrange the chicken in a single layer in the baking dish. Lightly spray the chicken with cooking spray.

3. Bake for 20–25 minutes, or until the chicken is no longer pink in the center and the top coating is slightly crisp.

Exchanges / Choices
1 Starch, 3 Lean Meat

Calories	200	Sodium	160 mg
Calories from Fat	35	Potassium	515 mg
Total Fat	**4 g**	**Total Carbohydrate**	**14 g**
Saturated Fat	1 g	Dietary Fiber	1 g
Trans Fat	0 g	Sugars	1 g
Polyunsaturated Fat	1 g	**Protein**	**26 g**
Monounsaturated Fat	1.5 g	**Phosphorus**	**300 mg**
Cholesterol	**70 mg**		

CHICKEN AND ASPARAGUS TOSS

Serves 4 / Serving Size: scant 1 cup chicken mixture and 1/2 cup rice

Juicy chicken and tender asparagus are cooked quickly and then bathed in a light, lemony sauce. A bed of brown rice soaks up all that citrusy goodness. Get an extra dose of lemon by serving Lemon-Raspberry Squares (page 169) for dessert.

1/2 cup uncooked instant brown rice

1 1/2 teaspoons grated lemon zest

2–3 tablespoons fresh lemon juice

2 tablespoons olive oil

1/2 teaspoon salt

6 ounces asparagus, trimmed and cut into 2-inch pieces

Cooking spray

1 pound boneless, skinless chicken breasts, all visible fat discarded, cut into bite-size pieces

1 1/2 teaspoons dried dillweed, crumbled

1 medium garlic clove, minced

1. Prepare the rice using the package directions, omitting the salt and margarine. Set aside.

2. Meanwhile, in a small bowl, whisk together the lemon zest, lemon juice, oil, and salt. Set aside.

3. In a large skillet, bring 1/2 cup water to a boil over high heat. Add the asparagus and return to a boil. Reduce the heat and simmer, covered, for 2 minutes, or until the asparagus is just tender-crisp. Drain well in a colander. Set aside.

4. Wipe the skillet with paper towels. Lightly spray the skillet with cooking spray. Cook the chicken and dillweed for 4 minutes, or until the chicken is no longer pink in the center, stirring frequently.

5. Stir the asparagus and garlic into the chicken mixture. Cook for 30 seconds, or until the asparagus is heated through, stirring constantly. Remove from the heat.

6. Add the lemon zest mixture to the chicken mixture, stirring gently to coat.

7. Spoon the rice onto a platter. Spoon the chicken mixture over the rice.

Exchanges / Choices
1 1/2 Starch, 4 Lean Meat

Calories	290	**Sodium**	330 mg
Calories from Fat	100	**Potassium**	600 mg
Total Fat	11 g	**Total Carbohydrate**	21 g
Saturated Fat	2 g	Dietary Fiber	2 g
Trans Fat	0 g	Sugars	1 g
Polyunsaturated Fat	1.5 g	**Protein**	27 g
Monounsaturated Fat	7 g	**Phosphorus**	330 mg
Cholesterol	70 mg		

CITRUS CHICKEN

Serves 4 / Serving Size: 3 ounces chicken and 2 tablespoons sauce

If one citrus juice is good, three must be terrific! The marinade for this chicken dish combines the brightness of grapefruit, orange, and lemon juices. Honey tames their tartness and fresh ginger and red pepper flakes add a spark of heat. Try serving the chicken over Toasted-Almond Rice and Peas (page 133) so none of the delicious sauce goes to waste.

1 cup 100% grapefruit juice (see Cook's Tip on page 24)

1/4 cup frozen 100% orange juice concentrate

2 tablespoons honey

1 tablespoon fresh lemon juice

2 teaspoons grated peeled gingerroot

1/8 teaspoon crushed red pepper flakes

4 boneless, skinless chicken breast halves (about 4 ounces each), all visible fat discarded

Cooking spray

1 tablespoon light tub margarine

1/4 teaspoon salt

1. In a medium glass bowl, whisk together the grapefruit juice, orange juice concentrate, honey, lemon juice, gingerroot, and red pepper flakes. Remove and set aside 1 cup of the juice mixture.

2. Add the chicken to the juice mixture remaining in the bowl, turning to coat. Cover and refrigerate for 15 minutes, turning once halfway through.

3. Lightly spray a large skillet with cooking spray. Heat over medium-high heat. Drain the chicken, discarding the marinade. Cook the chicken for 4 minutes. Turn over. Cook for 2–4 minutes, or until no longer pink in the center. Transfer to plates.

4. Stir the reserved 1 cup juice mixture into the pan residue. Increase the heat to high and bring to a boil. Boil for 3 minutes, or until the mixture is reduced by half (to about 1/2 cup), scraping to dislodge any browned bits. Remove from the heat.

5. Stir in the margarine and salt. Pour the sauce over the chicken.

Exchanges / Choices
1 Carbohydrate, 1/2 Fruit, 3 Lean Meat

Calories	230	Sodium	260 mg
Calories from Fat	40	Potassium	650 mg
Total Fat	4.5 g	Total Carbohydrate	22 g
Saturated Fat	1 g	Dietary Fiber	<1 g
Trans Fat	0 g	Sugars	20 g
Polyunsaturated Fat	1 g	Protein	25 g
Monounsaturated Fat	1.5 g	Phosphorus	260 mg
Cholesterol	70 mg		

SEARED CHICKEN WITH STRAWBERRY SALSA

Serves 4 / Serving Size: 3 ounces chicken and 1/2 cup salsa

Luscious strawberries are a different but delectable choice for this salsa, although you can substitute mango or peaches if you prefer. Whatever fruit you choose, the sweet and spicy salsa pairs perfectly with seared chicken breasts. Serve with mild sides to keep the flavor focus on this mealtime star. *(See photo insert.)*

1/2 teaspoon paprika

1/4 teaspoon ground allspice or cumin

1/4 teaspoon salt

1/4 teaspoon pepper

4 boneless, skinless chicken breast halves (about 4 ounces each), all visible fat discarded

Salsa

1 cup diced hulled strawberries, mango, or peeled peaches

1 medium poblano pepper, seeds and ribs discarded, diced, or 3/4 medium green bell pepper, diced

1/2 cup finely chopped red onion

1/4 cup chopped fresh mint or cilantro

2 tablespoons fresh lemon juice

1 tablespoon sugar

1/8 teaspoon crushed red pepper flakes

2 teaspoons canola or corn oil

1. In a small bowl, stir together the paprika, allspice, salt, and pepper. Sprinkle over the smooth side of the chicken. Using your fingertips, gently press the mixture so it adheres to the chicken. Let stand for 10 minutes.

2. Meanwhile, in a medium bowl, stir together the salsa ingredients.

3. In a large skillet, heat the oil over medium-high heat, swirling to coat the bottom. Cook the chicken with the smooth side down for 4 minutes. Turn over. Cook for 2–4 minutes, or until no longer pink in the center.

4. Serve the salsa with the chicken.

Exchanges / Choices	
1 Carbohydrate, 3 Lean Meat	

Calories	200	**Sodium**	230 mg
Calories from Fat	50	**Potassium**	590 mg
Total Fat	6 g	**Total Carbohydrate**	11 g
Saturated Fat	1 g	Dietary Fiber	1 g
Trans Fat	0 g	Sugars	6 g
Polyunsaturated Fat	1 g	**Protein**	25 g
Monounsaturated Fat	2.5 g	**Phosphorus**	255 mg
Cholesterol	70 mg		

SKILLET CHICKEN WITH LIME BARBECUE SAUCE

Serves 4 / Serving Size: 3 ounces chicken and 1 1/2 tablespoons sauce

Limeade adds an unusual, zesty tang to barbecue sauce. This chicken is cooked on the stovetop, so you can have a summery barbecue any time of year by adding some steamed green beans and Creamy Potato Salad (page 36).

Cooking spray

4 boneless, skinless chicken breast halves (about 4 ounces each), all visible fat discarded

1/4 cup barbecue sauce (lowest sodium available)

1/4 cup frozen limeade concentrate

1/4 teaspoon crushed red pepper flakes

1/2 teaspoon grated peeled gingerroot (optional)

1. Lightly spray a large skillet with cooking spray. Heat over medium-high heat. Cook the chicken for 4 minutes on each side, or until no longer pink in the center. Transfer to plates.

2. In a small bowl, stir together the barbecue sauce, limeade concentrate, and red pepper flakes. Stir into the pan juices. Cook for 1 minute, or until reduced slightly, stirring constantly and scraping to dislodge any browned bits. Remove from the heat.

3. Stir the gingerroot into the sauce. Spoon over the chicken.

Exchanges / Choices

1 Carbohydrate, 3 Lean Meat

Calories	200	**Sodium**	150 mg
Calories from Fat	30	**Potassium**	460 mg
Total Fat	3 g	**Total Carbohydrate**	18 g
Saturated Fat	1 g	Dietary Fiber	<1 g
Trans Fat	0 g	Sugars	16 g
Polyunsaturated Fat	0.5 g	**Protein**	24 g
Monounsaturated Fat	1 g	**Phosphorus**	240 mg
Cholesterol	70 mg		

SPANISH TACOS

Serves 4 / Serving Size: 2 tacos

Filled with shredded chicken simmered in mixed-vegetable juice seasoned with pungent turmeric, these tacos are a delicious alternative to the traditional Mexican version. A no-fuss green salad is all you need to complete the meal.

1 1/2 cups low-sodium mixed-vegetable juice

3 medium garlic cloves, minced

1/2 teaspoon ground turmeric

1/4 teaspoon salt

1/4 teaspoon pepper

4 boneless, skinless chicken breast halves (about 4 ounces each), all visible fat discarded, halved lengthwise

8 (6-inch) corn tortillas

1 medium tomato, seeded and diced

1/2 medium avocado, diced

1 1/4 ounces queso fresco, crumbled

1. In a medium nonstick skillet, stir together the juice, garlic, turmeric, salt, and pepper. Add the chicken. Bring to a boil over medium-high heat. Reduce the heat and simmer for 5 minutes. Turn the chicken over. Simmer for 5 minutes, or until the chicken is no longer pink in the center. Remove from the heat.

2. Let stand for about 2 minutes, or until the chicken is cool enough to handle. Transfer to a cutting board. Using two forks, shred the chicken. Return it to the skillet. Bring to a simmer over low heat.

3. Meanwhile, warm the tortillas using the package directions.

4. Spoon the chicken down the center of each tortilla. Top with the tomato, avocado, and queso fresco. Fold the sides of the tortillas over the filling.

Exchanges / Choices

2 Starch, 4 Lean Meat

Calories	320	**Sodium**	390 mg
Calories from Fat	80	**Potassium**	870 mg
Total Fat	9 g	**Total Carbohydrate**	30 g
Saturated Fat	2.5 g	Dietary Fiber	5 g
Trans Fat	0 g	Sugars	5 g
Polyunsaturated Fat	1.5 g	**Protein**	30 g
Monounsaturated Fat	3.5 g	**Phosphorus**	460 mg
Cholesterol	80 mg		

CHICKEN WITH COUNTRY GRAVY

Serves 4 / Serving Size: 3 ounces chicken and 2 tablespoons gravy

When you're looking for something soothing, this down-home chicken dish fits the bill. Pair it with low-fat mashed potatoes or a flavor-filled side, such as Green Beans with Mushrooms and Onions (page 136) or Brown-Sugar-and-Spice Sweet Potatoes (page 147).

3 tablespoons all-purpose flour

1 cup fat-free, low-sodium chicken broth

1/4 teaspoon paprika

1/4 teaspoon garlic powder

1/4 teaspoon poultry seasoning

Cooking spray

4 boneless, skinless chicken breast halves (about 4 ounces each), all visible fat discarded

2 tablespoons light tub margarine

1/4 teaspoon salt

1. Heat a large skillet over medium-high heat. Cook the flour for 1–2 minutes, or until beginning to lightly brown, stirring constantly with a flat spatula to prevent scorching. Remove from the heat. Spread on a plate to cool.

2. In a small bowl, whisk together the broth, paprika, garlic powder, poultry seasoning, and cooled flour.

3. Lightly spray the same skillet with cooking spray. Cook the chicken with the smooth side down for 2 minutes, or until beginning to brown. Transfer to a plate (the chicken won't be done at this point).

4. Reduce the heat to medium. Melt the margarine in the skillet, swirling to coat the bottom. Stir in the broth mixture, scraping to dislodge any browned bits.

5. Stir in the salt. Add the chicken. Spoon the gravy over the chicken. Reduce the heat and simmer, covered, for 10 minutes, or until the chicken is no longer pink in the center, stirring frequently.

6. Just before serving, transfer the chicken to a platter. Pour the gravy over the chicken.

Exchanges / Choices
1/2 Carbohydrate, 3 Lean Meat

Calories	190	Sodium	290 mg
Calories from Fat	50	Potassium	490 mg
Total Fat	6 g	Total Carbohydrate	6 g
Saturated Fat	1.5 g	Dietary Fiber	<1 g
Trans Fat	0 g	Sugars	0 g
Polyunsaturated Fat	1.5 g	Protein	26 g
Monounsaturated Fat	2 g	Phosphorus	260 mg
Cholesterol	70 mg		

CHICKEN STIR-FRY WITH SNOW PEAS AND MIXED BELL PEPPERS

Serves 4 / Serving Size: 3 ounces chicken and 3/4 cup vegetables

Bell peppers provide a rainbow of colors in this attractive stir-fry. The crispness of the peppers and snow peas contrasts with the juicy chunks of chicken, while a traditional stir-fry sauce bathes the dish in Asian flavors of soy, garlic, and ginger. Add brown rice for a meal that rivals your favorite from the Chinese takeout menu.

1/2 cup fat-free, low-sodium chicken broth

2 tablespoons plain rice vinegar

1 1/2 tablespoons soy sauce (lowest sodium available)

1 teaspoon grated peeled gingerroot

2 medium garlic cloves, minced

1/4 teaspoon pepper

Cooking spray

2 cups fresh or frozen snow peas or sugar snap peas, trimmed if fresh or thawed if frozen

1/3 cup chopped green onions

1/2 medium red bell pepper, chopped

1/2 medium green bell pepper, chopped

1/2 medium yellow bell pepper, chopped

2 teaspoons canola or corn oil

1 pound boneless, skinless chicken breasts, all visible fat discarded, cut into bite-size pieces

2 teaspoons cornstarch

1/4 cup water

1. In a small bowl, whisk together the broth, vinegar, soy sauce, gingerroot, garlic, and pepper. Set aside.

2. Lightly spray a large skillet or wok with cooking spray. Cook the snow peas, green onions, and all the bell peppers over medium-high heat for 4–5 minutes, or until tender-crisp, stirring occasionally. Transfer to a plate.

3. In the same skillet, heat the oil, swirling to coat the bottom. Cook the chicken for 4–5 minutes, or until no longer pink in the center, stirring frequently.

4. Return the snow pea mixture to the skillet. Stir in the broth mixture. Bring to a boil, still over medium-high heat. Boil for 1 minute, stirring occasionally.

5. Put the cornstarch in a small bowl. Add the water, stirring to dissolve. Stir into the chicken mixture. Cook for 45 seconds– 1 minute, or until thickened, stirring occasionally.

Exchanges / Choices
2 Vegetable, 3 Lean Meat

Calories	200	Sodium	370 mg
Calories from Fat	50	Potassium	660 mg
Total Fat	**6 g**	**Total Carbohydrate**	**9 g**
Saturated Fat	1 g	Dietary Fiber	2 g
Trans Fat	0 g	Sugars	3 g
Polyunsaturated Fat	1 g	**Protein**	**27 g**
Monounsaturated Fat	2.5 g	**Phosphorus**	**290 mg**
Cholesterol	**70 mg**		

DIJON CHICKEN WITH BROCCOLI AND NOODLES

Serves 5 / Serving Size: 2 1/2 ounces chicken, 1/2 cup sauce, and 1 cup broccoli and pasta

A rich, velvety mustard sauce blankets savory chicken tenders on a bed of noodles and tender-crisp broccoli—it's an all-in-one meal. Smoked paprika and cayenne add just a hint of smoky heat.

6 ounces dried whole-grain no-yolk noodles

2 1/2 cups chopped broccoli florets

3 tablespoons all-purpose flour

1 teaspoon smoked paprika

1/8 teaspoon cayenne

1 pound chicken tenders, all visible fat discarded

3 teaspoons olive oil, divided use

8 ounces sliced mushrooms, such as button, brown (cremini), portobello, or shiitake (stems discarded)

1 cup chopped onion

2 medium garlic cloves, minced

16 ounces fat-free plain Greek yogurt

3 tablespoons Dijon mustard (lowest sodium available)

1. Prepare the pasta using the package directions, omitting the salt. Three minutes before the end of the cooking time, stir in the broccoli. Drain in a colander. Set aside.

2. Meanwhile, in a medium shallow dish, stir together the flour, paprika, and cayenne. Dip the chicken in the flour mixture, turning to coat and shaking off any excess. Using your fingertips, gently press the coating mixture so it adheres to the chicken. Transfer to a large plate.

3. In a large nonstick skillet, heat 2 teaspoons oil over medium-high heat, swirling to coat the bottom. Cook the chicken for 4 minutes. Turn over. Cook for 2–4 minutes, or until no longer pink in the center. Transfer to a separate large plate. Cover loosely to keep warm.

4. Reduce the heat to medium. In the same skillet, heat the remaining 1 teaspoon oil, swirling to coat the bottom. Cook the mushrooms, onion, and garlic for 2–3 minutes, or until the onion begins to soften, stirring frequently and scraping to dislodge any browned bits. Remove from the heat.

5. Stir in the yogurt and mustard. Stir in the chicken. Serve over the pasta.

Cook's Tip on Greek Yogurt: Thicker and richer tasting than traditional yogurt, Greek yogurt is an excellent source of calcium, and a half-cup provides about the same amount of protein as 2 ounces of cooked meat.

Exchanges / Choices
2 Carbohydrate, 1 Vegetable, 4 Lean Meat

Calories	360	Sodium	150 mg
Calories from Fat	60	Potassium	890 mg
Total Fat	7 g	Total Carbohydrate	38 g
Saturated Fat	1.5 g	Dietary Fiber	3 g
Trans Fat	0 g	Sugars	7 g
Polyunsaturated Fat	1.5 g	Protein	36 g
Monounsaturated Fat	3.5 g	Phosphorus	480 mg
Cholesterol	100 mg		

CREOLE DRUMS

Serves 4 / Serving Size: 2 drumsticks and 1 cup vegetable mixture

Flavorful chicken legs are smothered in a Louisiana-style mixture of tomatoes, okra, onion, and bell pepper, and spiced up with hot-pepper sauce. Serve them in shallow soup bowls so you can easily spoon up all the great-tasting sauce or spoon them onto a bed of fluffy brown rice.

Cooking spray

8 skinless chicken drumsticks with bone, all visible fat discarded (about 2 pounds)

1 large onion, chopped

1 medium green bell pepper, chopped

1 (14.5-ounce) can no-salt-added diced tomatoes, undrained

10 ounces fresh or frozen cut okra, cut into 1/2-inch slices if fresh

1 teaspoon Worcestershire sauce (lowest sodium available)

1/2 teaspoon dried thyme, crumbled

1/4 teaspoon red hot-pepper sauce

1/8 teaspoon salt

1. Lightly spray a Dutch oven with cooking spray. Heat over medium-high heat. Cook the chicken for about 4 minutes, or until browned on all sides, turning frequently (the chicken won't be done at this point). Transfer to a plate.

2. In the same pot, cook the onion and bell pepper for 3 minutes, or until the edges are beginning to lightly brown, stirring frequently and scraping to dislodge any browned bits.

3. Gently stir in the chicken with any accumulated juices. Stir in the remaining ingredients except the salt. Bring to a boil, still over medium-high heat. Reduce the heat and simmer, covered, for 40 minutes, or until the chicken is no longer pink in the center and the okra is very tender. Remove from the heat.

4. Transfer the chicken to soup bowls. Stir the salt into the tomato mixture. Pour over the chicken.

Exchanges / Choices
3 Vegetable, 6 Lean Meat

Calories	330	Sodium	300 mg
Calories from Fat	60	Potassium	1400 mg
Total Fat	7 g	Total Carbohydrate	17 g
Saturated Fat	1.5 g	Dietary Fiber	4 g
Trans Fat	0 g	Sugars	10 g
Polyunsaturated Fat	1 g	Protein	51 g
Monounsaturated Fat	2 g	Phosphorus	560 mg
Cholesterol	150 mg		

CHICKEN PIZZA SAUTÉ

Serves 4 / Serving Size: 3/4 cup chicken mixture and 1/2 cup pasta

Opt for this creative one-dish meal when you crave the flavor of pizza but want something healthier. Whole-grain pasta shells are covered with a tomato sauce with fennel, garlic, and oregano. Mushrooms and ground chicken add substance, and the dish is topped off with a generous amount of fat-free mozzarella.

3 ounces dried medium whole-grain pasta shells (about 1 1/4 cups)

1 tablespoon olive oil

12 ounces ground skinless chicken breast

1 teaspoon fennel seeds, crushed

1 teaspoon dried oregano, crumbled

1 medium garlic clove, minced

8 ounces sliced mushrooms, such as button, brown (cremini), portobello, or shiitake (stems discarded)

1 medium bell pepper (any color), thinly sliced

1/2 medium red onion, thinly sliced

1 (14.5-ounce) can no-salt-added diced tomatoes, undrained

1/4 teaspoon salt

1/4 teaspoon pepper

1 cup shredded or grated fat-free mozzarella cheese

1. Prepare the pasta using the package directions, omitting the salt. Drain well in a colander. Cover to keep warm. Set aside.

2. Meanwhile, in a large nonstick skillet, heat the oil over medium heat, swirling to coat the bottom. Cook the chicken, fennel seeds, oregano, and garlic for 6–7 minutes, or until the chicken is almost cooked through, stirring occasionally to turn and break up the chicken.

3. Stir in the mushrooms, bell pepper, and onion. Cook for 5 minutes, or until the bell pepper is tender and the onion is soft, stirring occasionally.

4. Stir in the tomatoes with liquid, salt, and pepper. Bring to a simmer, and simmer for 5 minutes, stirring occasionally.

5. Spoon the pasta onto plates. Top with the chicken mixture. Sprinkle with the mozzarella.

Exchanges / Choices
2 Carbohydrate, 4 Lean Meat

Calories	320	Sodium	270 mg
Calories from Fat	100	Potassium	1140 mg
Total Fat	11 g	Total Carbohydrate	29 g
Saturated Fat	2.5 g	Dietary Fiber	5 g
Trans Fat	0 g	Sugars	7 g
Polyunsaturated Fat	2 g	Protein	30 g
Monounsaturated Fat	6 g	Phosphorus	505 mg
Cholesterol	80 mg		

CHICKEN POT PIE

Serves 6 / Serving Size: 1 1/2 cups

The whole-wheat crust for this bountiful dish is very easy to make—no rolling required! It's really more like a thick batter that's spread over the filling. Stick with the traditional combo of carrots, green beans, and corn, or branch out and try something unexpected.

Cooking spray

16 ounces unseasoned frozen mixed vegetables, any combination

2/3 cup fat-free, low-sodium chicken broth

2 teaspoons cornstarch

2 tablespoons water

1 pound chopped cooked chicken breast, cooked without salt, skin and all visible fat discarded

2/3 cup low-fat buttermilk

1 large egg

1 tablespoon trans-fat-free light stick margarine, melted and cooled

2/3 cup whole-wheat pastry flour

1/3 cup cornmeal

2 tablespoons minced fresh parsley

1 1/2 teaspoons baking powder

1/4 teaspoon salt

1. Preheat the oven to 425°F. Lightly spray an 11 x 7 x 2-inch glass baking dish with cooking spray.

2. In a medium saucepan, prepare the vegetables using the package directions, omitting the salt and margarine. Drain well in a colander. Set aside.

3. In the same saucepan, bring the broth to a boil over medium-high heat.

4. Put the cornstarch in a small bowl. Add the water, stirring to dissolve. Stir into the broth. Cook for 1 minute, or until the mixture comes to a boil and thickens, stirring frequently. Remove from the heat.

5. Stir in the chicken and vegetables. Pour into the baking dish.

6. In a medium bowl, whisk together the buttermilk, egg, and margarine. Stir in the remaining ingredients until just combined. Spread the batter over the chicken mixture.

7. Bake for 30–35 minutes, or until the crust is golden brown and a wooden toothpick inserted in the center of the crust comes out clean.

Exchanges / Choices

2 Starch, 4 Lean Meat

Calories	290	**Sodium**	380 mg
Calories from Fat	50	**Potassium**	510 mg
Total Fat	6 g	**Total Carbohydrate**	28 g
Saturated Fat	1.5 g	Dietary Fiber	4 g
Trans Fat	0 g	Sugars	5 g
Polyunsaturated Fat	0.5 g	**Protein**	31 g
Monounsaturated Fat	4 g	**Phosphorus**	355 mg
Cholesterol	95 mg		

ROAST TURKEY WITH ORANGE-SPICE RUB

Serves 11 / Serving Size: 3 ounces turkey

An aromatic spice rub cooks into a rich paste that penetrates deep into the turkey breast. Don't save this one for the holidays; it's great year-round. If you're lucky, you'll have turkey left over to use in Cranberry-Pecan Turkey Salad (page 40) or as an alternative for the chicken in Chicken Pot Pie (page 82).

Cooking spray

1 tablespoon grated orange zest

1/2 teaspoon ground cinnamon

1/2 teaspoon ground cumin

1/2 teaspoon paprika

1/4 teaspoon ground allspice, 1/4 teaspoon ground nutmeg, or 1/8 teaspoon ground cloves

1/4 teaspoon salt

1/4 teaspoon pepper

1/8 teaspoon cayenne

1 (5-pound) turkey breast with bone and skin

1. Preheat the oven to 325°F. Lightly spray a roasting pan and baking rack with cooking spray.

2. In a small bowl, stir together all the ingredients except the turkey.

3. Put the turkey on a cutting board or flat work surface. Carefully loosen the skin from the turkey breast by gently inserting your fingers between the skin and the meat, making a pocket for the orange zest mixture. Don't break the skin. Discard any fat beneath the skin. Still working carefully, spread the orange zest mixture under the loosened skin as well as possible. Transfer the turkey to the rack in the pan.

4. Roast the turkey for 1 hour 45 minutes, or until it registers 170°F–175°F on an instant-read thermometer inserted into the thickest part. Be sure the thermometer doesn't touch the bone. Remove the turkey from the oven.

5. Let the turkey stand for 15 minutes. Discard the skin and all visible fat before slicing.

Exchanges / Choices

3 Lean Meat

Calories	140	Sodium	120 mg
Calories from Fat	35	Potassium	260 mg
Total Fat	4 g	Total Carbohydrate	0 g
Saturated Fat	1 g	Dietary Fiber	0 g
Trans Fat	0 g	Sugars	0 g
Polyunsaturated Fat	1 g	Protein	25 g
Monounsaturated Fat	1 g	Phosphorus	180 mg
Cholesterol	65 mg		

TURKEY MARSALA

Serves 4 / Serving Size: 3 ounces turkey and 2 1/2 tablespoons sauce

Marsala is a fortified wine from Sicily with a distinctive, rich flavor that pairs well with poultry. Here, we lighten up the classic sauce with a bit of lemon and thyme. Try it on a bed of farro, whole-grain pasta, or Italian Skillet Spinach (page 143).

3 tablespoons cornstarch

1 teaspoon grated lemon zest

1 teaspoon dried thyme, crumbled

1/4 teaspoon pepper

1 pound boneless, skinless turkey breast, cut crosswise into 4 slices, or 1 pound turkey cutlets, all visible fat discarded

2 teaspoons canola or corn oil

1/3 cup dry marsala or dry red wine (regular or nonalcoholic)

1/3 cup fat-free, low-sodium chicken broth

2 tablespoons fresh lemon juice

2 tablespoons chopped fresh Italian (flat-leaf) parsley

1. In a small bowl, stir together the cornstarch, lemon zest, thyme, and pepper. Sprinkle over both sides of the turkey. Using your fingertips, gently press the mixture so it adheres to the turkey.

2. In a medium skillet, heat the oil over medium-high heat, swirling to coat the bottom. Cook the turkey for 3–4 minutes on each side, or until lightly browned and no longer pink in the center. Transfer the turkey to a platter. Cover to keep warm.

3. Increase the heat to high. In the same skillet, bring the marsala, broth, lemon juice, and parsley to a boil. Boil for 1 minute, or until the sauce is reduced slightly, scraping to dislodge any browned bits.

4. Spoon the sauce over the turkey.

Exchanges / Choices

1/2 Carbohydrate, 4 Lean Meat

Calories	210	Sodium	60 mg
Calories from Fat	35	Potassium	470 mg
Total Fat	**4 g**	**Total Carbohydrate**	**7 g**
Saturated Fat	1 g	Dietary Fiber	<1 g
Trans Fat	0 g	Sugars	0 g
Polyunsaturated Fat	0 g	**Protein**	**27 g**
Monounsaturated Fat	0 g	Phosphorus	270 mg
Cholesterol	**65 mg**		

STIR-FRY TURKEY WITH BROCCOLI AND MUSHROOMS

Serves 4 / Serving Size: 3 ounces turkey and 3/4 cup vegetables

A variety of fresh vegetables add crispness to this classic stir-fry, while pineapple adds a tart sweetness. Serve over brown rice or the whole grain of your choice.

3/4 cup 100% pineapple juice, divided use

2 tablespoons hoisin sauce (lowest sodium available)

1 teaspoon toasted sesame oil

1/2 teaspoon ground cardamom

1/4 teaspoon crushed red pepper flakes

Cooking spray

1 pound boneless, skinless turkey tenderloins, all visible fat discarded, cut into thin strips

1 1/2 teaspoons canola or corn oil

2 cups small broccoli florets

1 medium rib of celery, sliced

1/2 cup sliced green onions

1 1/2 cups sliced exotic mushrooms, such as straw, enoki, or wood ear, or button mushrooms

2 medium garlic cloves, minced

1 (8-ounce) can sliced water chestnuts, drained

2 teaspoons cornstarch

1. In a small bowl, whisk together 1/2 cup pineapple juice, hoisin sauce, sesame oil, cardamom, and red pepper flakes. Set aside.

2. Lightly spray a large skillet or wok with cooking spray. Heat over medium-high heat. Cook the turkey for 5–7 minutes, or until no longer pink in the center, stirring frequently. Transfer to a plate. Cover loosely to keep warm.

3. Reduce the heat to medium. In the same skillet, heat the canola oil, swirling to coat the bottom. Cook the broccoli, celery, and green onions for 3–4 minutes, or until the broccoli is tender-crisp, stirring frequently.

4. Stir in the mushrooms and garlic. Cook for 2–4 minutes, or until the mushrooms begin to soften.

5. Stir in the turkey, water chestnuts, and pineapple juice mixture. Increase the heat to medium high and bring to a boil.

6. Put the cornstarch in a small bowl. Add the remaining 1/4 cup pineapple juice, stirring to dissolve. Stir into the turkey mixture. Cook for 1 minute, or until the mixture comes to a boil and thickens, stirring frequently.

Cook's Tip: Water chestnuts grow underground and resemble muddy flower bulbs. A good source of fiber, water chestnuts add crunch to stir-fries, salads, and side dishes.

Exchanges / Choices
2 Vegetable, 1/2 Carbohydrate, 3 Lean Meat, 1 Fat

Calories	270	Sodium	170 mg
Calories from Fat	70	Potassium	840 mg
Total Fat	8 g	Total Carbohydrate	20 g
Saturated Fat	1 g	Dietary Fiber	3 g
Trans Fat	0 g	Sugars	8 g
Polyunsaturated Fat	2 g	Protein	30 g
Monounsaturated Fat	5 g	Phosphorus	370 mg
Cholesterol	65 mg		

TURKEY LOAF

Serves 4 / Serving Size: 2 slices

Serve this moist, vegetable-flecked meat loaf with Acorn Squash with Dried Apricots and Plums (page 144) for a colorful and delicious meal that can bake at the same time. If there are any leftovers, you can make great cold sandwiches on whole-grain bread or rolls.

Cooking spray

1 pound ground skinless extra-lean turkey breast

5/6 cup no-salt-added tomato sauce, divided use

1/2 cup diced onion

1 medium rib of celery, diced

1/2 medium red or green bell pepper, diced

1/3 cup finely crushed fat-free, unsalted whole-grain crackers

1 large egg

2 teaspoons balsamic or red wine vinegar

1/2 teaspoon dried thyme, crumbled

1/4 teaspoon salt

1/4 teaspoon pepper

1 1/2 teaspoons honey

1. Preheat the oven to 350°F. Lightly spray a broiler pan and rack or a roasting pan and baking rack with cooking spray.

2. In a large bowl, using your hands or a spoon, combine the turkey, 1/2 cup tomato sauce, the onion, celery, bell pepper, cracker crumbs, egg, vinegar, thyme, salt, and pepper. Shape into a loaf about 8 1/4 × 4 1/2 × 2 1/4 inches. Transfer it onto the rack in the pan. Bake for 55 minutes.

3. Meanwhile, in a small bowl, stir together the remaining 1/3 cup tomato sauce and the honey. Spread over the top of the turkey loaf.

4. Bake for 15–20 minutes, or until the loaf is cooked through and the topping is hot. Let stand for 5 minutes before cutting into slices.

Exchanges / Choices
1 Carbohydrate, 4 Lean Meat

Calories	220	**Sodium**	260 mg
Calories from Fat	30	**Potassium**	620 mg
Total Fat	**3 g**	**Total Carbohydrate**	**18 g**
Saturated Fat	1 g	Dietary Fiber	1 g
Trans Fat	0 g	Sugars	6 g
Polyunsaturated Fat	1 g	**Protein**	**30 g**
Monounsaturated Fat	1 g	**Phosphorus**	**320 mg**
Cholesterol	**110 mg**		

TURKEY CHILI

Serves 4 / Serving Size: 1 1/2 cups

Fresh jalapeño and crushed red pepper flakes, combined with meaty turkey breast and kidney beans, will get your attention. This chili will be the star of your table, with just a simple green salad and a crusty whole-grain roll on the side.

1 1/2 teaspoons canola or corn oil

1/2 cup chopped red onion

2 medium garlic cloves, minced

1 teaspoon ground cumin

1 teaspoon dried oregano, crumbled

1 teaspoon chopped fresh jalapeño, seeds and ribs discarded

1/4 teaspoon crushed red pepper flakes

1 pound ground skinless extra-lean turkey breast

1 (14.5-ounce) can no-salt-added diced tomatoes, undrained

1 (8-ounce) can no-salt-added tomato sauce

1 cup fat-free, low-sodium chicken broth

1 (15.5-ounce) can no-salt-added kidney beans, rinsed and drained

1. In a medium nonstick saucepan, heat the oil over medium heat, swirling to coat the bottom. Cook the onion and garlic for about 2 minutes, or until tender-crisp, stirring frequently.

2. Stir in the cumin, oregano, jalapeño, and red pepper flakes. Cook for 1 minute, stirring constantly.

3. Increase the heat to medium high. Stir in the turkey. Cook for 3–4 minutes, or until browned on the outside, stirring occasionally to turn and break up the turkey.

4. Stir in the remaining ingredients. Bring to a boil, still over medium-high heat. Reduce the heat and simmer, partially covered, for 30 minutes, or until the liquid is reduced by about one-third.

Exchanges / Choices
2 Starch, 4 Lean Meat

Calories	330	Sodium	130 mg
Calories from Fat	30	Potassium	1290 mg
Total Fat	**3.5 g**	**Total Carbohydrate**	**41 g**
Saturated Fat	1 g	Dietary Fiber	10 g
Trans Fat	0 g	Sugars	10 g
Polyunsaturated Fat	1 g	**Protein**	**37 g**
Monounsaturated Fat	1.5 g	**Phosphorus**	**460 mg**
Cholesterol	**70 mg**		

| *Meats* |

MUSTARD-CRUSTED
BEEF TENDERLOIN

Serves 8 / Serving Size: 3 ounces beef

The high heat of the oven sears the mustard crust onto the succulent beef in this impressive entrée, locking in the juices. While the beef is resting, reduce the oven temperature a bit and cook Pecan-Roasted Asparagus (page 132) for a delectable side dish.

Cooking spray

3 tablespoons country Dijon or coarse-grain mustard (lowest sodium available)

2 tablespoons chopped fresh thyme or 2 teaspoons dried thyme, crumbled

4 medium garlic cloves, minced

1/2 teaspoon salt

1/2 teaspoon pepper

1 (2-pound) beef tenderloin, all visible fat and silver skin discarded

1. Preheat the oven to 450°F. Lightly spray a shallow roasting pan with cooking spray.

2. In a small bowl, whisk together the mustard, thyme, garlic, salt, and pepper.

3. Put the beef in the pan. Spread the mustard mixture over the beef.

4. Roast for 25–30 minutes, or to the desired doneness. Transfer to a cutting board. Cover the beef loosely with aluminum foil. Let stand for 10–15 minutes.

5. Just before serving, thinly slice the beef diagonally across the grain.

Cook's Tip: The tough membrane sometimes found on the outside of tenderloin and flank steak is called silver skin. It should be discarded before the beef is cooked. Slide a sharp knife under the silver skin and cut it off. Leaving the silver skin on will cause the beef to curl up during cooking.

Exchanges / Choices
4 Lean Meat

Calories	180	**Sodium**	250 mg
Calories from Fat	70	**Potassium**	400 mg
Total Fat	8 g	**Total Carbohydrate**	0 g
Saturated Fat	3 g	Dietary Fiber	0 g
Trans Fat	0 g	Sugars	0 g
Polyunsaturated Fat	0.5 g	**Protein**	25 g
Monounsaturated Fat	3 g	**Phosphorus**	235 mg
Cholesterol	75 mg		

SLOW-COOKER MEDITERRANEAN POT ROAST

Serves 8 / Serving Size: 3 ounces beef, 1/3 cup sauce, and 1 cup pasta

Beef is at its tender best after being simmered with pasta sauce and Italian spices, then nestled on a bed of whole-grain spaghetti. The slow cooker does most of the work, too—including enticing everyone to the table with the savory aroma.

2 teaspoons dried basil, crumbled

3 medium garlic cloves, minced

1 teaspoon dried oregano, crumbled

1/2 teaspoon salt

1/4 teaspoon crushed red pepper flakes

1 (2 1/2-pound) boneless top round steak or boneless chuck roast, all visible fat discarded, cut to fit in the slow cooker, if necessary

1 1/2 cups spaghetti sauce, such as tomato basil (lowest sodium available), divided use

16 ounces dried whole-grain spaghetti

1. In a small bowl, stir together the basil, garlic, oregano, salt, and red pepper flakes. Sprinkle over both sides of the beef. Using your fingertips, gently press the mixture so it adheres to the beef.

2. Pour 1 cup spaghetti sauce into a 3- to 4 1/2-quart round or oval slow cooker. Place the beef on the sauce. Pour the remaining 1/2 cup sauce over the beef. Cook, covered, on low for 7–8 hours, or until the beef is fork-tender. Transfer to a cutting board. Cover the beef loosely with aluminum foil. Skim off and discard any fat from the sauce in the slow cooker.

3. About 15 minutes before serving time, prepare the pasta using the package directions, omitting the salt. Drain well in a colander.

4. Thinly slice the beef diagonally across the grain. Arrange the pasta on plates. Place the beef on the pasta. Ladle the sauce over all.

Cook's Tip: If the roast is too wide to fit into your slow cooker, halve it crosswise and stack it.

Exchanges / Choices
3 Starch, 4 Lean Meat

Calories	390	Sodium	160 mg
Calories from Fat	45	Potassium	780 mg
Total Fat	5 g	Total Carbohydrate	47 g
Saturated Fat	2 g	Dietary Fiber	6 g
Trans Fat	0 g	Sugars	5 g
Polyunsaturated Fat	1 g	Protein	41 g
Monounsaturated Fat	2 g	Phosphorus	445 mg
Cholesterol	75 mg		

ROAST SIRLOIN AND VEGETABLE SUPPER

Serves 8 / Serving Size: 3 ounces beef and 1 cup vegetables

Sometimes, nothing satisfies like a juicy steak along with potatoes and carrots. Shallots and fennel add both bite and a mild sweetness to our version of the classic comfort-food combo. Creamy Caramelized Onion Soup (page 14) makes a soothing starter and complements the beefy flavors.

Cooking spray

1 (2-pound) boneless top sirloin steak, about 1 1/2 inches thick, all visible fat discarded

2 pounds red potatoes, cut into 1-inch pieces

8 ounces baby carrots

8 ounces medium shallots or large pearl onions, peeled

1 large fennel bulb or 1 large turnip, cut into 1/2-inch-thick wedges

1 cup fat-free, low-sodium beef broth

2 teaspoons dried thyme, crumbled

2 teaspoons paprika

1 teaspoon dried oregano, crumbled

3/4 teaspoon salt

1/2 teaspoon dried minced garlic or garlic powder

1/2 teaspoon dried rubbed sage, crumbled

1/2 teaspoon pepper

1. Preheat the oven to 350°F. Lightly spray a large shallow roasting pan with cooking spray.

2. Put the beef in the center of the pan. Arrange the potatoes, carrots, shallots, and fennel around the beef. Pour the broth over the vegetables.

3. In a small bowl, stir together the remaining ingredients. Sprinkle over the beef and vegetables.

4. Roast for 40–45 minutes, or until the beef is the desired doneness. Transfer the beef to a cutting board. Cover loosely with aluminum foil. Let stand for 10 minutes.

5. Meanwhile, stir the vegetables. Using the tip of a sharp knife, test the vegetables for tenderness. Roast for 5–10 minutes, or until tender, if needed.

6. Thinly slice the beef diagonally across the grain. Transfer to plates. Arrange the vegetables around the beef. Spoon any pan juices over all.

Exchanges / Choices

1 1/2 Starch, 1 Vegetable, 3 Lean Meat

Calories	280	Sodium	290 mg
Calories from Fat	45	Potassium	1320 mg
Total Fat	**5 g**	**Total Carbohydrate**	**29 g**
Saturated Fat	1.5 g	Dietary Fiber	5 g
Trans Fat	0 g	Sugars	5 g
Polyunsaturated Fat	0.5 g	**Protein**	**30 g**
Monounsaturated Fat	2 g	**Phosphorus**	**375 mg**
Cholesterol	**80 mg**		

MUSHROOM-SMOTHERED CUBE STEAK

Serves 4 / Serving Size: 3 ounces beef and 1/3 cup mushroom sauce

Reminiscent of chicken-fried steak, this easy-on-the-cook main dish is blanketed with mushroom sauce instead of cream gravy. Add a side of colorful steamed vegetables and serve the beef over brown rice or quinoa to soak up the sauce.

1/2 teaspoon salt

1/2 teaspoon pepper

4 cube steaks (about 4 ounces each), all visible fat discarded

2 tablespoons all-purpose flour

3 teaspoons canola or corn oil, divided use

1/3 cup chopped shallots or sweet onion, such as Vidalia, Maui, or Oso Sweet

8 ounces sliced mushrooms, such as button, brown (cremini), portobello, or shiitake (stems discarded)

2 medium garlic cloves, minced

1/2 cup fat-free, low-sodium beef broth

1. Preheat the oven to 200°F.

2. Sprinkle the salt and pepper over the beef.

3. Put the flour in a shallow dish or bowl. Dredge the beef in the flour, patting and turning until all the flour adheres to the beef.

4. In a large nonstick skillet, heat 2 teaspoons oil over medium-high heat, swirling to coat the bottom. Cook the beef for 3 minutes on each side, or until golden brown on the outside and still pink in the center.

5. Transfer the beef to an ovenproof platter. Cover with aluminum foil. Put the platter in the oven.

6. In the same skillet, heat the remaining 1 teaspoon oil over medium-high heat, swirling to coat the bottom. Reduce the heat to medium. Cook the shallots for 2 minutes, stirring occasionally.

7. Stir in the mushrooms and garlic. Cook for 5 minutes, stirring occasionally.

8. Stir in the broth. Reduce the heat and simmer for 5 minutes, or until the sauce thickens, stirring occasionally.

9. Just before serving, transfer the beef to plates. Spoon the sauce over the beef.

Cook's Tip: Cube steaks are thin, boneless top sirloin or top or bottom round steaks that have been tenderized on a cubing machine, a piece of equipment used by butchers to tenderize meat and bind smaller pieces of meat into steaks. The machine leaves cube-shaped markings on the surface of the meat.

Exchanges / Choices
1 Vegetable, 4 Lean Meat, 1/2 Fat

Calories	220	Sodium	410 mg
Calories from Fat	70	Potassium	670 mg
Total Fat	**8 g**	**Total Carbohydrate**	**6 g**
Saturated Fat	2.5 g	Dietary Fiber	1 g
Trans Fat	0 g	Sugars	1 g
Polyunsaturated Fat	1 g	**Protein**	**28 g**
Monounsaturated Fat	4.5 g	**Phosphorus**	**300 mg**
Cholesterol	**60 mg**		

FABULOUS FAJITAS

Serves 6 / Serving Size: 1 fajita

These beef fajitas, with their savory Tex-Mex spices, will put some sizzle in your evening meal. Fiesta Slaw (page 30) makes a tempting accompaniment, or make it a party by serving Layered Fiesta Bean Dip (page 2) as a starter.

1 (1 1/2-pound) flank steak, all visible fat and silver skin discarded

1/4 cup fresh lime juice

3 medium garlic cloves, minced

Cooking spray

2 teaspoons chili powder

2 teaspoons ground cumin

2 teaspoons ground coriander

1/4 teaspoon cayenne

2 large bell peppers (1 red and 1 green preferred), halved, stemmed, and seeds and ribs discarded

2 (1/4-inch-thick) slices from 1 large white or red onion

6 (8-inch) fat-free whole-wheat tortillas (lowest sodium available)

1/4 cup plus 2 tablespoons salsa (lowest sodium available)

1/4 cup plus 2 tablespoons chopped fresh cilantro

1. Put the beef in a shallow glass dish. Sprinkle the lime juice and garlic over the beef. Cover and refrigerate for 30 minutes–2 hours, turning occasionally.

2. When the beef is marinated, lightly spray the grill rack or a broiler pan and rack with cooking spray. Preheat the grill on medium high or preheat the broiler.

3. In a small bowl, stir together the chili powder, cumin, coriander, and cayenne.

4. Drain the beef, discarding the marinade and leaving the garlic clinging to the beef. Transfer to a flat surface, such as a large baking sheet. Place the bell pepper halves and onion slices on the baking sheet. Lightly spray with cooking spray. Sprinkle the chili powder mixture over both sides of the beef, bell peppers, and onion. Using your fingertips, gently press the chili powder mixture so it adheres to the beef and vegetables. (The spray helps the mixture adhere to the vegetables.)

5. Grill the beef, bell peppers, and onion or broil them about 5 inches from the heat for 6 minutes. Turn them over. Grill or broil for 5–6 minutes, or until the vegetables are tender and the beef is the desired doneness. Transfer the beef and vegetables to a cutting board.

6. Cover the beef loosely with aluminum foil. Let stand for 5 minutes. Meanwhile, cut the bell peppers into 1/4-inch strips. Separate the onion slices into rings. Thinly slice the beef diagonally across the grain.

7. Warm the tortillas using the package directions.

8. Place the beef and vegetables down the center of the tortillas. Top with the salsa and cilantro. Fold the sides of the tortillas over the filling.

Cook's Tip: Make a double batch of the chili powder mixture so you'll have extra to keep on hand. Sprinkle some on lean beef or chicken before grilling, or add some to tomato soup for deep, rich flavor and color.

Exchanges / Choices

2 Starch, 1 Vegetable, 3 Lean Meat

Calories	310	**Sodium**	340 mg
Calories from Fat	35	**Potassium**	680 mg
Total Fat	4 g	**Total Carbohydrate**	39 g
Saturated Fat	1.5 g	Dietary Fiber	2 g
Trans Fat	0 g	Sugars	4 g
Polyunsaturated Fat	0.5 g	**Protein**	31 g
Monounsaturated Fat	1.5 g	**Phosphorus**	320 mg
Cholesterol	60 mg		

SPICY ORANGE FLANK STEAK

Serves 4 / Serving Size: 3 ounces beef

Tangy orange melds beautifully with robust garlic, spicy red pepper flakes, and briny soy sauce in this grilled beef entrée. Throw some portobello mushrooms or asparagus on the grill as a simple and tasty side dish, or start your meal with Crunchy Asian Snow Pea Salad (page 28).

2 teaspoons grated orange zest, divided use

1/4 cup fresh orange juice

2 tablespoons soy sauce (lowest sodium available)

3 medium garlic cloves, minced

1/2 teaspoon crushed red pepper flakes

1 (1-pound) flank steak, all visible fat and silver skin discarded

Cooking spray

1. In a large shallow glass dish, whisk together 1 teaspoon orange zest, the orange juice, soy sauce, garlic, and red pepper flakes. Add the beef, turning to coat. Cover and refrigerate for 30 minutes–2 hours, turning occasionally.

2. When the beef is marinated, lightly spray the grill rack with cooking spray. Preheat the grill on medium high.

3. Meanwhile, drain the beef, pouring the marinade into a small saucepan. Bring the marinade to a boil over high heat. Boil for at least 5 minutes. (This destroys harmful bacteria.)

4. Place the beef on the grill. Brush with the marinade. Grill, covered, for 4–5 minutes on each side for medium rare, or until the desired doneness. Transfer to a cutting board.

5. Lightly cover the beef with aluminum foil. Let stand for 5 minutes. Thinly slice diagonally across the grain.

6. Just before serving, sprinkle the beef with the remaining 1 teaspoon orange zest.

Exchanges / Choices
4 Lean Meat

Calories	190	**Sodium**	380 mg
Calories from Fat	80	**Potassium**	480 mg
Total Fat	9 g	**Total Carbohydrate**	4 g
Saturated Fat	3.5 g	Dietary Fiber	<1 g
Trans Fat	0 g	Sugars	2 g
Polyunsaturated Fat	0.5 g	**Protein**	25 g
Monounsaturated Fat	4 g	**Phosphorus**	250 mg
Cholesterol	80 mg		

GRILLED SIRLOIN WITH TAPENADE

Serves 6 / Serving Size: 3 ounces beef and 1 heaping tablespoon tapenade

The pungent flavor of olives and capers accentuates the beefiness of grilled sirloin, which tastes best with simple sides such as grilled vegetables and brown rice or farro that let the steak take center stage.

Cooking spray

1 1/2 pounds boneless top sirloin steak, about 1 inch thick, all visible fat discarded

4 1/2 medium garlic cloves, minced

1 1/2 teaspoons dried thyme, crumbled

1/2 teaspoon pepper

1/8 teaspoon salt

Tapenade

1/4 cup chopped kalamata olives

3 tablespoons chopped pimiento-stuffed green olives

1 tablespoon Dijon mustard (lowest sodium available)

1 tablespoon capers, drained, and chopped if large

1/2 teaspoon dried thyme, crumbled

1/2 medium garlic clove, minced

1. Lightly spray the grill rack with cooking spray. Preheat the grill on medium high.

2. Lightly spray the beef with cooking spray.

3. In a small bowl, stir together the garlic cloves, thyme, pepper, and salt. Sprinkle over the beef. Using your fingertips, gently press the mixture so it adheres to the beef.

4. Grill the beef, covered, for 10 minutes on each side for medium rare, or until the desired doneness. Transfer to a cutting board. Lightly cover with aluminum foil. Let stand for 5 minutes. Thinly slice the beef diagonally across the grain.

5. Meanwhile, in a separate small bowl, stir together the tapenade ingredients.

6. Serve the beef topped with the tapenade.

Cook's Tip: The word tapenade comes from *tapeno*, the Provençal word for capers. This multipurpose paste is made of capers, olives, garlic, and, usually, anchovies and olive oil. It is usually very high in sodium, so use it sparingly.

Exchanges / Choices
4 Lean Meat

Calories	180	Sodium	300 mg
Calories from Fat	60	Potassium	400 mg
Total Fat	**7 g**	**Total Carbohydrate**	**2 g**
Saturated Fat	2.5 g	Dietary Fiber	1 g
Trans Fat	0 g	Sugars	0 g
Polyunsaturated Fat	0.5 g	**Protein**	**26 g**
Monounsaturated Fat	4 g	**Phosphorus**	**225 mg**
Cholesterol	**60 mg**		

SLOW-COOKER SWISS STEAK

Serves 6 / Serving Size: 3 ounces beef, 2/3 cup sauce, and scant 1 cup noodles

A slow cooker braises top round steak to tender perfection in this melt-in-your-mouth dish. The name is not a reference to Switzerland; instead it refers to the process of "swissing," or tenderizing the meat by pounding it with a meat mallet or heavy pan.

2 tablespoons all-purpose flour

1 teaspoon dried basil, crumbled

1 teaspoon dried oregano, crumbled

1/2 teaspoon salt

1/2 teaspoon pepper

1 1/2 pounds boneless top round steak, all visible fat discarded, cut into 6 pieces

1 medium onion, thinly sliced

3 medium garlic cloves, thinly sliced

1 medium green bell pepper, cut into 3/4-inch squares

1 1/2 cups spaghetti sauce, such as tomato basil (lowest sodium available)

8 ounces dried whole-grain no-yolk noodles

1 teaspoon balsamic vinegar

2 tablespoons chopped fresh basil

1. In a small bowl, stir together the flour, dried basil, oregano, salt, and pepper.

2. Sprinkle half the flour mixture over one side of the beef. Using the smooth side of a meat mallet or a heavy pan, pound the flour into the beef. Turn over. Repeat with the remaining flour mixture, pounding until all of it is absorbed into the beef.

3. Put the onion in a 3- to 4 1/2-quart round or oval slow cooker. Place the beef on the onion. Sprinkle the garlic and then the bell pepper over the beef. Pour the spaghetti sauce over all. Cook, covered, on low for 8 hours or on high for 4 hours, or until the beef is fork-tender.

4. About 15 minutes before serving time, prepare the pasta using the package directions, omitting the salt. Drain well in a colander. Transfer the pasta to plates.

5. Place the beef on the pasta. Stir the vinegar into the sauce in the slow cooker. Spoon the sauce over the beef and pasta. Sprinkle with the fresh basil.

Exchanges / Choices

2 1/2 Starch, 1 Vegetable, 3 Lean Meat

Calories	350	**Sodium**	230 mg
Calories from Fat	50	**Potassium**	810 mg
Total Fat	6 g	**Total Carbohydrate**	40 g
Saturated Fat	2 g	Dietary Fiber	3 g
Trans Fat	0 g	Sugars	8 g
Polyunsaturated Fat	1 g	**Protein**	33 g
Monounsaturated Fat	2 g	**Phosphorus**	360 mg
Cholesterol	100 mg		

SPICY BEEF AND ONION KEBABS

Serves 4 / Serving Size: 1 kebab

These wonderfully zesty kebabs are perfect for the grilling season. Fresh summer corn on the cob sprinkled with lemon pepper can grill right alongside the kebabs for an equally flavorful side dish.

1/4 cup beer (light or nonalcoholic)

1/4 cup no-salt-added ketchup

3 medium garlic cloves, minced

1 teaspoon dry mustard

1 teaspoon red hot-pepper sauce

1/2 teaspoon salt

1 pound boneless top sirloin steak, about 1 1/4 inches thick, all visible fat discarded, cut into 16 cubes

Cooking spray

1 large onion, cut through the core into 16 wedges, each about 1/3 inch thick

1. In a large shallow glass dish, whisk together the beer, ketchup, garlic, mustard, hot-pepper sauce, and salt. Add the beef, turning to coat. Cover and refrigerate for 30 minutes–2 hours, turning occasionally.

2. When the beef is marinated, lightly spray the grill rack with cooking spray. Preheat the grill on medium high.

3. Drain the beef, pouring the marinade into a small saucepan. Bring the marinade to a boil over high heat. Boil for at least 5 minutes. (This destroys harmful bacteria.)

4. Alternately thread 4 beef cubes and 4 onion wedges onto each of four metal skewers.

5. Place the kebabs on the grill. Brush with half the marinade.

6. Grill, covered, for 5 minutes. Turn over the kebabs. Using a clean basting brush, brush with the remaining marinade. Grill, covered, for 5–8 minutes for medium rare, or until the beef is the desired doneness.

Cook's Tip: Cutting the onion through the core keeps the wedges attached by the root, making it easier to thread them onto the skewers.

Exchanges / Choices
2 Vegetable, 3 Lean Meat, 1/2 Fat

Calories	210	Sodium	310 mg
Calories from Fat	50	Potassium	540 mg
Total Fat	**6 g**	**Total Carbohydrate**	**11 g**
Saturated Fat	2.5 g	Dietary Fiber	1 g
Trans Fat	0 g	Sugars	8 g
Polyunsaturated Fat	0.5 g	**Protein**	**26 g**
Monounsaturated Fat	3 g	**Phosphorus**	**255 mg**
Cholesterol	**60 mg**		

SIRLOIN AND BROCCOLI STIR-FRY

Serves 4 / Serving Size: 1 cup stir-fry and 1/2 cup rice

This fragrant dish pairs classic Asian seasonings with an unusual mixture of vegetables, including red cabbage and summer squash, all of which complement the beef. Served over nutty-tasting brown rice, this all-in-one meal provides protein, vegetables, and a whole grain. *(See photo insert.)*

1 tablespoon cornstarch

1 tablespoon soy sauce (lowest sodium available)

1 teaspoon grated peeled gingerroot

1 medium garlic clove, minced

1 pound boneless sirloin steak, all visible fat discarded, cut crosswise into 1/4-inch strips, longer strips halved crosswise

1 cup uncooked instant brown rice

1 cup fat-free, low-sodium beef broth

2 tablespoons hoisin sauce (lowest sodium available)

1 teaspoon toasted sesame oil

1 teaspoon canola or corn oil

3 ounces broccoli florets, broken into bite-size pieces

1 medium yellow summer squash, thinly sliced crosswise

4 medium green onions, thinly sliced

2 ounces red cabbage, shredded

1–2 tablespoons water (as needed)

1. Put the cornstarch in a medium bowl. Add the soy sauce, gingerroot, and garlic, whisking to dissolve the cornstarch. Add the beef, turning to coat. Cover and refrigerate for 10 minutes, turning occasionally.

2. Meanwhile, prepare the rice using the package directions, omitting the salt and margarine. Set aside.

3. In a small bowl, whisk together the broth, hoisin sauce, and sesame oil. Set aside.

4. In a large nonstick skillet or wok, heat the canola oil over medium-high heat, swirling to coat the bottom. Cook the beef mixture for 5 minutes, or until the beef is browned on the outside (it may be slightly pink in the center), stirring constantly. Transfer the beef mixture to a large plate.

5. In the same skillet, still over medium-high heat, stir together the remaining ingredients except the water. Cook for 2–3 minutes, or until the vegetables are tender-crisp, stirring constantly. If the mixture becomes too dry, stir in the water.

6. Return the beef mixture to the skillet. Pour in the broth mixture, stirring to combine. Cook for 1–2 minutes, or until the broth mixture thickens, stirring occasionally. Serve the stir-fry over the rice.

Exchanges / Choices
3 Starch, 4 Lean Meat

Calories	400	Sodium	380 mg
Calories from Fat	80	Potassium	780 mg
Total Fat	**9 g**	**Total Carbohydrate**	**47 g**
Saturated Fat	2.5 g	Dietary Fiber	4 g
Trans Fat	0 g	Sugars	4 g
Polyunsaturated Fat	2 g	**Protein**	**32 g**
Monounsaturated Fat	4 g	Phosphorus	410 mg
Cholesterol	**60 mg**		

BEEF TAGINE

Serves 4 / Serving Size: heaping 1 cup beef mixture and 1/2 cup couscous

This quick-cooking version of tagine, a Moroccan meat and vegetable dish slow-simmered with warm spices and served over couscous, uses cubes of tender steak that are browned, then reheated in the slightly sweet stew.

2 teaspoons olive oil

1 pound boneless sirloin steak, all visible fat discarded, cut into 1/2-inch cubes

1 large red bell pepper and 1 large yellow bell pepper, or 2 large red bell peppers, chopped

1 small onion, chopped

2 medium garlic cloves, minced

1/2 teaspoon ground ginger

1/2 teaspoon ground cumin

1/4 teaspoon salt

1/8 teaspoon ground allspice

1/8 teaspoon ground cinnamon

1 (14.5-ounce) can no-salt-added diced tomatoes, undrained

1 cup fat-free, low-sodium chicken broth

1/3 cup golden raisins

2 tablespoons no-salt-added tomato paste

1 cup uncooked whole-wheat couscous

2 tablespoons fresh lemon juice

1 tablespoon chopped fresh parsley

1. In a large skillet, heat the oil over medium-high heat, swirling to coat the bottom. Cook the beef for 3 minutes, or just until browned on all sides, stirring frequently. Transfer to a large plate. Set aside.

2. In the same skillet, still over medium-high heat, stir together the bell peppers, onion, and garlic. Cook for 5 minutes, stirring frequently.

3. Stir in the ginger, cumin, salt, allspice, and cinnamon. Cook for 1 minute, or until the spices are fragrant, stirring constantly.

4. Stir in the tomatoes with liquid, broth, raisins, and tomato paste. Bring to a boil. Reduce the heat and simmer, covered, for 12–15 minutes, or until the bell peppers and onion are very tender, with no crispness remaining.

5. Meanwhile, prepare the couscous using the package directions, omitting the salt. Fluff with a fork.

6. Stir the beef into the bell pepper mixture. Cook for 1 minute, or just until the beef is heated through. Remove from the heat. Stir in the lemon juice and parsley. Serve the tagine over the couscous.

Exchanges / Choices
2 Starch, 3 Vegetable, 1 Fruit, 3 Lean Meat

Calories	440	Sodium	210 mg
Calories from Fat	50	Potassium	1150 mg
Total Fat	**6 g**	**Total Carbohydrate**	**62 g**
Saturated Fat	2 g	Dietary Fiber	6 g
Trans Fat	0 g	Sugars	16 g
Polyunsaturated Fat	1 g	**Protein**	**35 g**
Monounsaturated Fat	3.5 g	**Phosphorus**	**405 mg**
Cholesterol	**60 mg**		

TEX-MEX CHILI BOWL

Serves 4 / Serving Size: 1 1/4 cups

This hearty chili packs plenty of meaty flavor in every bowl, thanks to cubes of lean beef and a boost from broth. A dollop of creamy fat-free sour cream and a sprinkle of mild queso fresco add a cooling touch.

Cooking spray

12 ounces boneless top round or lean chuck steak, all visible fat discarded, cut into 3/4-inch cubes

1 medium onion, chopped

4 medium garlic cloves, minced

1 tablespoon chili powder

2 teaspoons ground cumin

1/4 teaspoon cayenne

1 cup fat-free, low-sodium beef broth

2 (15.5-ounce) cans no-salt-added pinto or black beans, or one of each, rinsed and drained

1 (14.5-ounce) can no-salt-added diced tomatoes, undrained

1/2 cup salsa or picante sauce (lowest sodium available)

1/4 cup fat-free sour cream

2 tablespoons crumbled queso fresco

1/4 cup chopped fresh cilantro

1. Lightly spray a large saucepan with cooking spray. Heat over medium-high heat. Cook the beef, onion, and garlic for 5 minutes, stirring frequently.

2. Stir in the chili powder, cumin, and cayenne. Cook for 1 minute, stirring frequently.

3. Pour in the broth. Increase the heat to high and bring to a boil. Reduce the heat and simmer, covered, for 1 hour, or until the beef is fork-tender, stirring once halfway through.

4. Stir in the beans, tomatoes with liquid, and salsa. Simmer, covered, for 10 minutes.

5. Serve the chili topped with the sour cream, queso fresco, and cilantro.

Cook's Tip: Queso fresco is a tangy Mexican cheese that crumbles easily and softens but does not melt. Check larger supermarkets and specialty markets for queso fresco, but if you don't find it, try crumbled farmer cheese, soft goat cheese, fat-free feta cheese, or shredded low-fat Monterey Jack.

Exchanges / Choices
2 Starch, 3 Vegetable, 4 Lean Meat

Calories	370	**Sodium**	400 mg
Calories from Fat	50	**Potassium**	1240 mg
Total Fat	**6 g**	**Total Carbohydrate**	**44 g**
Saturated Fat	1.5 g	Dietary Fiber	13 g
Trans Fat	0 g	Sugars	6 g
Polyunsaturated Fat	0.5 g	**Protein**	**35 g**
Monounsaturated Fat	1.5 g	**Phosphorus**	430 mg
Cholesterol	**50 mg**		

MEXICAN-STYLE STUFFED BELL PEPPERS

Serves 4 / Serving Size: 1 stuffed bell pepper

In this Latin twist on stuffed bell peppers, black beans replace the traditional rice and salsa stands in for the standard tomato sauce. *(See photo insert.)*

4 large red or green bell peppers, or a combination, stems, seeds, and ribs discarded, tops chopped and reserved

Cooking spray

1/2 cup chopped onion

3 medium garlic cloves, minced

8 ounces 95% fat-free ground beef

2 teaspoons chili powder

1 teaspoon ground cumin

1/8 teaspoon salt

3/4 cup salsa (lowest sodium available)

1 cup canned no-salt-added black beans, rinsed and drained

1/2 cup plus 2 tablespoons chopped fresh cilantro, divided use

1/4 cup low-fat shredded 4-cheese Mexican blend

1/4 cup fat-free sour cream

1. Preheat the oven to 375°F.

2. In a microwave oven, place the bell peppers with the cut side up on a paper towel. Microwave on 100% power (high) for 4–5 minutes, or until tender-crisp. Transfer with the cut side up to a 9-inch square baking dish or shallow casserole dish.

3. Meanwhile, lightly spray a large skillet with cooking spray. Heat over medium heat. Cook the chopped bell pepper tops, onion, and garlic for 5 minutes, stirring occasionally.

4. Stir in the beef. Cook for 5 minutes, stirring occasionally to turn and break up the beef. Discard any drippings.

5. Sprinkle the beef mixture with the chili powder, cumin, and salt. Cook for 1 minute. Stir in the salsa. Remove from the heat.

6. Gently stir in the beans and 1/2 cup cilantro. Spoon the beef mixture into the peppers. Cover the baking dish with aluminum foil.

7. Bake for 30 minutes, or until heated through. Remove from the oven. Sprinkle the Mexican blend cheese over the beef mixture. Let stand for 5 minutes.

8. Top the peppers with the sour cream. Sprinkle with the remaining 2 tablespoons cilantro.

Exchanges / Choices

1/2 Starch, 3 Vegetable, 2 Lean Meat, 1/2 Fat

Calories	230	Sodium	560 mg
Calories from Fat	50	Potassium	820 mg
Total Fat	**5 g**	**Total Carbohydrate**	**25 g**
Saturated Fat	2 g	Dietary Fiber	7 g
Trans Fat	0 g	Sugars	7 g
Polyunsaturated Fat	0.5 g	**Protein**	**21 g**
Monounsaturated Fat	2 g	**Phosphorus**	**290 mg**
Cholesterol	**40 mg**		

GRILLED MEAT LOAF

Serves 4 / Serving Size: 2 slices

This dish is a fresh alternative to boring burgers, with a deep, meaty flavor and a pleasantly crisp crust. Grill some asparagus or zucchini at the same time for a flavorful side dish, and add Creamy Potato Salad (page 36) to make your next backyard barbecue an affair to remember.

Cooking spray

1 slice whole-grain bread (lowest sodium available)

1 pound 95% fat-free ground beef

1/3 cup minced onion

1 large egg white

1/4 cup no-salt-added ketchup, divided use

1 medium garlic clove, minced

1/4 teaspoon salt

1/4 teaspoon pepper

1 tablespoon coarse-grain or Dijon mustard (lowest sodium available)

1. Lightly spray the grill rack with cooking spray. Preheat the grill on medium high.

2. Meanwhile, in a food processor or blender, process the bread into crumbs. Pour the crumbs into a medium bowl.

3. Using your hands or a spoon, combine the beef, onion, egg white, 2 tablespoons ketchup, the garlic, salt, and pepper with the bread crumbs. Shape into a 1 1/2-inch-thick oval patty.

4. Grill the meat loaf, covered, for 10 minutes. Using two spatulas, carefully turn over the meat loaf.

5. Meanwhile, in a small bowl, whisk to-gether the remaining 2 tablespoons ketchup and the mustard. Spread over the top of the meat loaf.

6. Grill, covered, for 10 minutes, or until the meat loaf registers 160°F on an instant-read thermometer and is no longer pink in the center.

7. Remove from the grill. Let stand for 5 minutes before cutting into slices.

Cook's Tip: You can process extra whole-grain bread crumbs and freeze them in airtight plastic freezer bags for up to two months.

Exchanges / Choices
1/2 Carbohydrate, 4 Lean Meat

Calories	210	**Sodium**	280 mg
Calories from Fat	50	**Potassium**	500 mg
Total Fat	6 g	**Total Carbohydrate**	9 g
Saturated Fat	2.5 g	Dietary Fiber	1 g
Trans Fat	0 g	Sugars	4 g
Polyunsaturated Fat	0.5 g	**Protein**	27 g
Monounsaturated Fat	2.5 g	**Phosphorus**	255 mg
Cholesterol	70 mg		

HAM AND BROCCOLI FRITTATA

Serves 4 / Serving Size: 1/4 frittata

Serve this tasty egg dish with a salad of mixed greens and some seasonal fresh fruit when you need to get supper on the table in a hurry. It's also delicious for brunch.

Cooking spray

2 cups frozen fat-free potatoes O'Brien, thawed

6 ounces small broccoli florets, rinsed in cold water, drained, but not dried (some water droplets should cling to the broccoli)

8 large egg whites

1 large egg

4 ounces lower-sodium, low-fat ham, cut into 1/4-inch cubes

1/4 cup fat-free milk

1/4 teaspoon pepper

1. Preheat the oven to 400°F.

2. Lightly spray a medium ovenproof skillet with cooking spray. Heat over medium heat. Remove from the heat. Put the potatoes in the skillet. Lightly spray with cooking spray. Cook for 4–5 minutes, or until the potatoes are golden brown, stirring occasionally.

3. Put the broccoli in a microwaveable bowl. Microwave, covered, on 100% power (high) for 3–4 minutes, or until tender-crisp. Drain in a colander. Stir the broccoli into the potatoes.

4. In a medium bowl, whisk together the egg whites and egg. Whisk in the ham, milk, and pepper. Pour the mixture over the potatoes and broccoli, stirring well.

5. Bake for 15–18 minutes, or until the eggs are set (don't jiggle when the frittata is gently shaken).

Cook's Tip: If your skillet is not ovenproof, wrap the handle in heavy aluminum foil before putting it in the oven.

Exchanges / Choices
1 Carbohydrate, 2 Lean Meat

Calories	180	**Sodium**	460 mg
Calories from Fat	30	**Potassium**	570 mg
Total Fat	3 g	**Total Carbohydrate**	17 g
Saturated Fat	1 g	Dietary Fiber	2 g
Trans Fat	0 g	Sugars	4 g
Polyunsaturated Fat	0.5 g	**Protein**	18 g
Monounsaturated Fat	1.5 g	**Phosphorus**	210 mg
Cholesterol	60 mg		

ASIAN BARBECUED PORK TENDERLOIN

Serves 4 / Serving Size: 3 ounces pork

Traditional Asian barbecued pork is slowly smoked and gets its bright red hue from food coloring. This easy version gets its beautiful color and tangy taste from a mixture of hickory barbecue sauce and Asian flavors.

Marinade

2 tablespoons hickory barbecue sauce (lowest sodium available)

1 tablespoon soy sauce (lowest sodium available)

1 tablespoon plain rice vinegar or cider vinegar

2 medium garlic cloves, minced

1 teaspoon minced peeled gingerroot

1/2 teaspoon Szechuan peppercorns, crushed, or 1/4 teaspoon crushed red pepper flakes

1 (1-pound) pork tenderloin, all visible fat discarded

Cooking spray

1/4 cup water

1. In a large glass baking dish, whisk together the marinade ingredients. Add the pork, turning to coat. Cover and refrigerate for 30 minutes–2 hours, turning occasionally.

2. When the pork is marinated, lightly spray the grill rack or broiler pan and rack with cooking spray. Preheat the grill on medium high or preheat the broiler.

3. Drain the pork, pouring the marinade into a small saucepan. Stir in the water. Bring to a boil over high heat. Boil for at least 5 minutes. (This destroys harmful bacteria.)

4. Place the pork on the grill or broiler rack. Brush with half the marinade. Grill, covered, or broil about 4–5 inches from the heat for 8 minutes. Turn over. Using a clean basting brush, brush with the remaining marinade. Grill, covered, or broil for 8 minutes. Turn over. Grill, covered, or broil for 2–4 minutes, or until the pork registers 145°F on an instant-read thermometer. Transfer to a cutting board.

5. Lightly cover the pork with aluminum foil. Let stand for 3 minutes before cutting crosswise into thin slices.

Exchanges / Choices
3 Lean Meat

Calories	140	**Sodium**	440 mg
Calories from Fat	30	**Potassium**	630 mg
Total Fat	**3 g**	**Total Carbohydrate**	**4 g**
Saturated Fat	1 g	Dietary Fiber	<1 g
Trans Fat	0 g	Sugars	3 g
Polyunsaturated Fat	0.5 g	**Protein**	**24 g**
Monounsaturated Fat	1 g	**Phosphorus**	340 mg
Cholesterol	**50 mg**		

SOUTHWESTERN PORK TENDERLOIN SKILLET

Serves 4 / Serving Size: 2 pork medallions and 3/4 cup hominy mixture

This one-skillet pork dish showcases vibrant south-of-the-border flavors, including spicy chili powder and cayenne, smoky cumin, chewy hominy, and tender corn. Add a tropical fruit salad, such as Caribbean Fruit Salad Platter (page 34), and let the fiesta begin.

2 teaspoons chili powder

1 teaspoon ground cumin

1/8 teaspoon cayenne

1 (1-pound) pork tenderloin, all visible fat discarded, cut crosswise into 8 slices, each slice flattened to 1/2-inch thickness (for medallions)

1 teaspoon canola or corn oil

1 medium green bell pepper, cut into 1/2-inch squares

1/2 (15-ounce) can white hominy, rinsed and drained

1 1/2 cups frozen whole-kernel corn, thawed

1/2 cup salsa (lowest sodium available)

2 tablespoons chopped fresh cilantro or green onions, thinly sliced (green part only)

1. In a small bowl, stir together the chili powder, cumin, and cayenne. Remove and set aside 1/2 teaspoon of the mixture. Sprinkle the remaining chili powder mixture over both sides of the pork. Using your fingertips, gently press the mixture so it adheres to the pork.

2. In a large nonstick skillet, heat the oil over medium-high heat, swirling to coat the bottom. Cook the pork for 3 minutes. Reduce the heat to medium. Turn over the pork. Cook for 3 minutes (the pork won't be done at this point). Transfer to a plate. Set aside.

3. In the same skillet, still over medium heat, cook the bell pepper for 5 minutes, stirring occasionally. Stir in the hominy, corn, salsa, and reserved chili powder mixture. Cook for 3 minutes, or until the bell pepper is tender.

4. Return the pork and any accumulated juices to the skillet. Cook for 4 minutes, or until the pork registers 145°F on an instant-read thermometer, turning once halfway through. Remove from the heat. Let stand for 3 minutes.

5. Just before serving, sprinkle with the cilantro.

Exchanges / Choices
1 1/2 Starch, 3 Lean Meat

Calories	230	Sodium	420 mg
Calories from Fat	45	Potassium	700 mg
Total Fat	4.5 g	Total Carbohydrate	21 g
Saturated Fat	1 g	Dietary Fiber	4 g
Trans Fat	0 g	Sugars	5 g
Polyunsaturated Fat	1.5 g	Protein	26 g
Monounsaturated Fat	2 g	Phosphorus	340 mg
Cholesterol	70 mg		

SPICY PORK CHOPS WITH SWEET MANGO SAUCE

Serves 4 / Serving Size: 1 pork chop and 1/3 cup sauce

You can almost feel the island breezes when you savor this Jamaican-inspired dish. Serve over fluffy brown rice or quinoa to catch all the fruit-filled sauce, with a side of Down-Home Greens (page 138).

Cooking spray

1 teaspoon paprika

1 teaspoon dried thyme, crumbled

1/8 teaspoon ground allspice

1/8 teaspoon cayenne

1/2 teaspoon salt

4 boneless pork loin chops, about 1/2 inch thick (about 4 ounces each), all visible fat discarded

1 tablespoon apricot all-fruit spread or pineapple preserves

1 medium mango, diced

2 tablespoons chopped fresh cilantro

1 tablespoon fresh lime juice

1. Lightly spray the grill rack with cooking spray. Preheat the grill on medium high.

2. In a small bowl, stir together the paprika, thyme, allspice, and cayenne. Remove and set aside 1/4 teaspoon of the mixture. Sprinkle the salt and remaining paprika mixture over the pork. Using your fingertips, gently press the seasonings so they adhere to the pork. Lightly spray with cooking spray.

3. Grill the pork, covered, for 5 minutes on each side, or until it registers 145°F on an instant-read thermometer. Remove from the grill. Let stand for 3 minutes.

4. Meanwhile, in a medium bowl, using a fork, briskly stir the apricot spread until softened. Stir in the mango, cilantro, lime juice, and reserved paprika mixture.

5. Serve the pork topped with the sauce.

Cook's Tip: If the preserves are very cold, soften them by microwaving them on 100% power (high) for 15 seconds, or let them stand at room temperature for 5 minutes before stirring.

Exchanges / Choices
1 Fruit, 3 Lean Meat

Calories	190	Sodium	280 mg
Calories from Fat	35	Potassium	520 mg
Total Fat	4 g	Total Carbohydrate	12 g
Saturated Fat	1 g	Dietary Fiber	1 g
Trans Fat	0 g	Sugars	9 g
Polyunsaturated Fat	0.5 g	Protein	27 g
Monounsaturated Fat	1.5 g	Phosphorus	295 mg
Cholesterol	70 mg		

ONION-SMOTHERED PORK CHOPS

Serves 4 / Serving Size: 1 pork chop and 1/4 cup onion

This hearty dish is ready in less than 30 minutes. Redolent with the homey aromas of sage and sautéed onions, it's an ideal comfort food when teamed with low-fat mashed potatoes and steamed green beans.

1 teaspoon paprika

1 teaspoon dried sage or thyme, crumbled

1/4 teaspoon salt

1/4 teaspoon pepper

4 boneless center-cut pork chops, about 1/2 inch thick (about 4 ounces each), all visible fat discarded

Cooking spray

2 large yellow or sweet onions, such as Vidalia, Maui, or Oso Sweet, thinly sliced, separated into rings

1/4 cup fat-free, low-sodium chicken broth, divided use

1 tablespoon Dijon mustard (lowest sodium available)

1. In a small bowl, stir together the paprika, sage, salt, and pepper. Sprinkle over the pork. Using your fingertips, gently press the mixture so it adheres to the pork.

2. Lightly spray a large skillet with cooking spray. Heat over medium heat. Cook the pork for 4 minutes on each side (the pork won't be done at this point). Transfer to a plate. Set aside.

3. In the same skillet, still over medium heat, cook the onions and 1 tablespoon broth, covered, for 5 minutes, stirring frequently. Cook, uncovered, for 5 minutes, or until the onions are golden brown, stirring once halfway through.

4. Stir in the remaining 3 tablespoons broth and the mustard. Return the pork to the skillet, placing it on the onions. Cook for 5 minutes, or until the onions are tender and the pork registers 145°F on an instant-read thermometer. Remove from the heat. Let stand for 3 minutes.

5. Transfer the pork to plates. Spoon the onions over the pork.

Exchanges / Choices
2 Vegetable, 3 Lean Meat

Calories	200	Sodium	280 mg
Calories from Fat	30	Potassium	630 mg
Total Fat	**3 g**	**Total Carbohydrate**	**13 g**
Saturated Fat	1 g	Dietary Fiber	2 g
Trans Fat	0 g	Sugars	8 g
Polyunsaturated Fat	0.5 g	**Protein**	**28 g**
Monounsaturated Fat	1.5 g	**Phosphorus**	**335 mg**
Cholesterol	**70 mg**		

THYME-SCENTED PORK CHOP AND BEAN SKILLET

Serves 4 / Serving Size: 3 pork strips and scant 1 cup beans

Ready in less than 30 minutes, this pork-and-beans dish is a lifesaver when you're short on time. The dried thyme adds a subtle woodsy flavor to the pork that balances the sweetness of the sauce. All you need add is a salad or some steamed vegetables.

1 teaspoon paprika

1 teaspoon dried thyme, crumbled

1/4 teaspoon salt

1/4 teaspoon pepper

3 boneless pork loin chops (about 4 ounces each), all visible fat discarded

Cooking spray

1/4 cup no-salt-added ketchup

2 tablespoons light brown sugar

1 tablespoon Dijon or spicy brown mustard (lowest sodium available)

1 tablespoon Worcestershire sauce (lowest sodium available)

1 (15.5-ounce) can no-salt-added kidney beans, drained and rinsed

1 (15.5-ounce) can no-salt-added pinto beans, drained and rinsed

1. In a small bowl, stir together the paprika, thyme, salt, and pepper. Sprinkle over both sides of the pork. Using your fingertips, gently press the mixture so it adheres to the pork.

2. Lightly spray a large skillet with cooking spray. Heat over medium-high heat. Cook the pork for 3 minutes on each side (the pork won't be done at this point). Transfer to a cutting board. Cut each pork chop into 4 strips. Set aside.

3. Stir the ketchup, brown sugar, mustard, and Worcestershire sauce together in the skillet. Reduce the heat to medium.

4. Stir in the kidney and pinto beans. Bring to a simmer. Reduce the heat and simmer for 5 minutes.

5. Return the pork to the skillet. Increase the heat to medium. Cook for 2 minutes on each side, or until the pork registers 145°F on an instant-read thermometer. Remove from the heat. Let stand for 3 minutes.

Cook's Tip: The combination of no-salt-added ketchup, brown sugar, Dijon mustard, and Worcestershire sauce creates a barbecue-type sauce. Prepare an extra batch. Cover and refrigerate it for up to one week. You don't need to cook the sauce before using it.

Exchanges / Choices
2 Starch, 1/2 Carbohydrate, 3 Lean Meat

Calories	330	**Sodium**	270 mg
Calories from Fat	35	**Potassium**	1100 mg
Total Fat	4 g	**Total Carbohydrate**	40 g
Saturated Fat	1 g	Dietary Fiber	14 g
Trans Fat	0 g	Sugars	9 g
Polyunsaturated Fat	0.5 g	**Protein**	31 g
Monounsaturated Fat	1.5 g	**Phosphorus**	420 mg
Cholesterol	60 mg		

| *Vegetarian Entrées* |

ROASTED-VEGGIE PIZZA ON A PHYLLO CRUST

Serves 6 / Serving Size: 1/6 pizza

A colorful variety of fresh vegetables nests on flaky phyllo dough, then is topped with just the right amount of cheese. Roasting brings out the sweetness of the veggies, packing the pizza with so much flavor that no sauce is needed.

Olive oil cooking spray

3 cups tightly packed spinach

12 ounces small broccoli florets

12 ounces asparagus, trimmed, cut into 2-inch pieces

6 ounces thickly sliced mushrooms, such as button, brown (cremini), portobello, or shiitake (stems discarded)

1 medium bell pepper (any color), chopped

1/2 cup chopped red onion

1/4 teaspoon pepper

6 14 × 9-inch frozen phyllo sheets, thawed

1/3 cup shredded low-fat mozzarella cheese

1/4 cup shredded or grated Parmesan cheese

1/4 teaspoon dried oregano or dried basil, crumbled

1/8 teaspoon crushed red pepper flakes

1. Preheat the oven to 425°F. Lightly spray a large baking dish with cooking spray.

2. Arrange the spinach, broccoli, asparagus, mushrooms, bell pepper, and onion in a single layer in the dish. Lightly spray the vegetables with cooking spray. Sprinkle with the pepper. Roast for 10–15 minutes, or until the onion is tender-crisp. Transfer the vegetables to a plate.

3. Wipe the baking dish with paper towels. Lightly spray the dish with cooking spray. Reduce the oven temperature to 400°F.

4. Keeping the unused phyllo covered with a damp cloth or damp paper towels to prevent drying, place 1 sheet in the pan. Lightly spray with cooking spray. Repeat with the remaining phyllo, layering each sheet on top of the previous one.

5. Spread the roasted vegetables over the layered phyllo. Sprinkle with the remaining ingredients.

6. Bake for 10–15 minutes, or until the mozzarella and Parmesan have melted and the crust is golden brown around the edges.

Cook's Tip on Phyllo: These fragile, paper-thin sheets of dough are usually found in the freezer section of the supermarket, near the piecrusts and puff pastry. Phyllo is made primarily of flour and water, with a small amount of oil and, possibly, some lemon juice. When baked, the dough becomes flaky and crumbly.

Exchanges / Choices

1/2 Starch, 3 Vegetable, 1 Fat

Calories	140	**Sodium**	220 mg
Calories from Fat	30	**Potassium**	560 mg
Total Fat	3.5 g	**Total Carbohydrate**	20 g
Saturated Fat	1.5 g	Dietary Fiber	4 g
Trans Fat	0 g	Sugars	4 g
Polyunsaturated Fat	0 g	**Protein**	8 g
Monounsaturated Fat	1 g	**Phosphorus**	180 mg
Cholesterol	5 mg		

SIX-INGREDIENT LASAGNA

Serves 6 / Serving Size: one 4 × 2 1/2-inch or 4 1/2 × 3-inch piece

This luscious and healthy dish is bursting with cheese and the flavors of Italy, and with so few ingredients, it's a snap to prepare. For a savory starter, try Salad Greens with Mixed-Herb Vinaigrette (page 25) or Italian Salsa Salad (page 31).

4 dried whole-grain lasagna noodles

1 (25.5-ounce) jar spaghetti sauce, such as roasted garlic or tomato basil (lowest sodium available)

1/4 teaspoon crushed red pepper flakes (optional)

1 (15-ounce) container fat-free ricotta cheese

1/4 cup plus 1 tablespoon chopped fresh basil, divided use

1 cup shredded low-fat mozzarella cheese, divided use

1. Prepare the noodles using the package directions, omitting the salt. Drain well in a colander. Set aside.

2. Preheat the oven to 375°F.

3. In a large skillet, stir together the spaghetti sauce and red pepper flakes. Bring to a simmer over medium-high heat. Reduce the heat and simmer for 5 minutes, stirring occasionally.

4. In a medium bowl, stir together the ricotta and 2 tablespoons basil.

5. In an 8- or 9-inch square baking dish, layer as follows: 3/4 cup sauce, 2 noodles, half the ricotta mixture, 1/2 cup mozzarella, 3/4 cup sauce, 2 noodles, the remaining ricotta mixture, and the remaining sauce. Cover with aluminum foil.

6. Bake for 40 minutes. Top with the remaining 1/2 cup mozzarella. Bake for 15 minutes, or until bubbly. Remove from the oven. Sprinkle with the remaining 3 tablespoons basil. Let stand for 5 minutes before cutting into pieces.

Exchanges / Choices

2 Vegetable, 1 Starch, 2 Lean Meat, 1 Fat

Calories	220	Sodium	240 mg
Calories from Fat	45	Potassium	620 mg
Total Fat	**5 g**	**Total Carbohydrate**	**25 g**
Saturated Fat	1.5 g	Dietary Fiber	3 g
Trans Fat	0 g	Sugars	11 g
Polyunsaturated Fat	0.5 g	**Protein**	**16 g**
Monounsaturated Fat	0.5 g	**Phosphorus**	**280 mg**
Cholesterol	**25 mg**		

EGGPLANT RICOTTA LASAGNA

Serves 4 / Serving Size: one 4-inch square

There's nothing like taking the eggplant from eggplant Parmesan and importing it into lasagna—what an inspired and delectable concept! This rich and hearty lasagna is sure to please vegetarians and carnivores alike.

4 1/2 dried whole-grain lasagna noodles

Cooking spray

8 ounces chopped unpeeled eggplant

1 small zucchini, cut crosswise into slices

1 large onion, chopped

2 medium garlic cloves, minced

2 cups no-salt-added tomato sauce

1 tablespoon plus 1 teaspoon dried basil, crumbled

3/4 tablespoon dried oregano, crumbled

1 cup fat-free ricotta cheese

1/4 teaspoon salt

1/2 cup shredded low-fat mozzarella cheese

1/4 cup shredded or grated Parmesan cheese

1. Prepare the noodles using the package directions, omitting the salt. Drain well in a colander. Set aside.

2. Meanwhile, preheat the oven to 350°F. Lightly spray an 8-inch square baking dish with cooking spray.

3. Lightly spray a large skillet with cooking spray. Heat over medium-high heat. Remove from the heat. Put the eggplant, zucchini, onion, and garlic in the skillet. Lightly spray with cooking spray. Cook for 6–7 minutes, or until the zucchini is just tender, stirring frequently. Remove from the heat. Set aside.

4. In a small bowl, stir together the tomato sauce, basil, and oregano.

5. Halve the 4 whole noodles crosswise. Place 3 noodle halves in one layer in the baking dish. Spread 2/3 cup tomato sauce mixture over the noodles. Using a teaspoon, dot 1/2 cup ricotta cheese over the sauce. Spoon 1 cup of the eggplant mixture over all. Sprinkle with half the salt. Repeat. Top with the final 3 noodle halves. Spoon the remaining sauce over all. Sprinkle with the mozzarella.

6. Bake for 30 minutes. Remove from the oven. Sprinkle with the Parmesan. Let stand for 15 minutes before cutting into squares.

Exchanges / Choices

4 Vegetable, 1 1/2 Carbohydrate, 2 Lean Meat

Calories	280	**Sodium**	420 mg
Calories from Fat	45	Potassium	950 mg
Total Fat	5 g	**Total Carbohydrate**	43 g
Saturated Fat	2.5 g	Dietary Fiber	8 g
Trans Fat	0 g	Sugars	17 g
Polyunsaturated Fat	0.5 g	**Protein**	17 g
Monounsaturated Fat	0.5 g	Phosphorus	350 mg
Cholesterol	30 mg		

SQUASH STUFFED WITH BULGUR AND ROASTED BELL PEPPERS

Serves 4 / Serving Size: 2 stuffed squash halves

Brimming with flavor, these tender squash boats are piled high with nutty bulgur, savory onion, and smoky-sweet roasted red bell pepper, and then topped with plenty of low-fat sharp cheddar cheese.

Cooking spray

1 cup uncooked instant, or fine-grain, bulgur

4 medium yellow summer squash or zucchini

1 1/2 large onions, chopped

1 tablespoon dried basil, crumbled

1 medium garlic clove, minced

1/4 teaspoon crushed red pepper flakes

8 ounces roasted red bell peppers (drained if bottled), chopped

1/2 cup chopped fresh parsley

1/8 teaspoon salt

3/4 cup shredded low-fat sharp cheddar cheese

1. Preheat the oven to 350°F. Lightly spray a 13 × 9 × 2-inch baking dish with cooking spray.

2. Prepare the bulgur using the package directions, omitting the salt. Fluff with a fork. Set aside.

3. Meanwhile, halve the squash lengthwise. Scoop out the pulp, leaving a 1/4-inch border of the shell all the way around. Place the squash shells with the cut side up in the baking dish. Set aside. Coarsely chop the pulp.

4. Lightly spray a large skillet with cooking spray. Heat over medium-high heat. Cook the onions for 4 minutes, or until tender, stirring frequently.

5. Stir in the chopped squash, basil, garlic, and red pepper flakes. Cook for 5 minutes, or until the squash is tender, stirring frequently. Remove from the heat. Stir in the bulgur, roasted peppers, parsley, and salt.

6. Spoon about 1/2 cup bulgur mixture into each of the squash shells. Using your fingertips or a spoon, firmly press the mixture down. Cover the dish with aluminum foil.

7. Bake for 30 minutes, or until the shells are tender. Sprinkle with the cheddar. Bake for 5 minutes, or until the cheddar has melted. Remove from the oven. Let stand for 5 minutes.

Exchanges / Choices

2 Vegetable, 2 Starch

Calories	220	Sodium	300 mg
Calories from Fat	30	Potassium	690 mg
Total Fat	**3 g**	**Total Carbohydrate**	**39 g**
Saturated Fat	1 g	Dietary Fiber	3 g
Trans Fat	0 g	Sugars	7 g
Polyunsaturated Fat	0.5 g	**Protein**	**9 g**
Monounsaturated Fat	1 g	**Phosphorus**	**205 mg**
Cholesterol	**5 mg**		

MIDDLE EASTERN BULGUR AND VEGETABLES

Serves 4 / Serving Size: 1/2 cup bulgur and 2/3 cup vegetable mixture

Tender, mildly sweet raisins balance nicely with crunchy pine nuts and warm spices in this aromatic dish that takes just minutes to prepare. It matches well with a simple salad of cucumbers and tomatoes or a Greek salad.

1 cup uncooked instant, or fine-grain, bulgur

Cooking spray

1 1/2 large onions, chopped

1 medium red bell pepper, chopped

6 ounces soy crumbles, thawed if frozen

1/3 cup pine nuts, dry-roasted

1/4 cup raisins

1/2 teaspoon ground cinnamon

1/4 teaspoon ground allspice, ground nutmeg, or ground cumin

1/4 teaspoon crushed red pepper flakes

1/8 teaspoon salt

Exchanges / Choices
2 Starch, 2 Vegetable, 2 Lean Meat, 1 Fat

Calories	350	Sodium	320 mg
Calories from Fat	110	Potassium	740 mg
Total Fat	12 g	Total Carbohydrate	52 g
Saturated Fat	1 g	Dietary Fiber	11 g
Trans Fat	0 g	Sugars	14 g
Polyunsaturated Fat	4 g	Protein	14 g
Monounsaturated Fat	2.5 g	Phosphorus	220 mg
Cholesterol	0 mg		

1. Prepare the bulgur using the package directions, omitting the salt. Fluff with a fork. Set aside.

2. Meanwhile, lightly spray a large skillet with cooking spray. Heat over medium-high heat. Remove from the heat. Put the onions and bell pepper in the skillet. Lightly spray with cooking spray. Cook for 6 minutes, or until the vegetables begin to richly brown, stirring frequently.

3. Stir in the remaining ingredients. Cook for 1 minute, or until the onion mixture is heated through.

4. Spoon the bulgur onto a platter. Top with the onion mixture.

SPINACH, ARTICHOKE, AND MUSHROOM TOSS

Serves 4 / Serving Size: 1 cup vegetable mixture and 1/2 cup quinoa

To step up a midweek meal, try this easy skillet dish. It's loaded with vegetables, topped with tangy feta, and served over hot, fluffy quinoa. *(See photo insert.)*

1/2 cup uncooked quinoa, rinsed and drained

Cooking spray

1 large onion, chopped

8 ounces sliced mushrooms, such as button, brown (cremini), portobello, or shiitake (stems discarded)

2 medium garlic cloves, minced

1 teaspoon dried oregano, crumbled

1/8 teaspoon crushed red pepper flakes

9 ounces frozen artichoke hearts, thawed and coarsely chopped

2 ounces coarsely chopped spinach

1/3 cup chopped roasted red bell peppers, drained if bottled

4 ounces fat-free feta cheese, crumbled

1/4 cup chopped fresh parsley

1. Prepare the quinoa using the package directions, omitting the salt. Fluff with a fork. Set aside.

2. Meanwhile, lightly spray a large skillet with cooking spray. Heat over medium-high heat. Cook the onion for 4 minutes, or until beginning to brown slightly on the edges, stirring frequently.

3. Stir in the mushrooms, garlic, oregano, and red pepper flakes. Remove from the heat. Lightly spray with cooking spray. Cook for 6 minutes, or until the mushrooms begin to lightly brown, stirring frequently.

4. Stir in the artichokes, spinach, and roasted peppers. Cook for 1 minute, or until the mixture is hot and the spinach begins to release its moisture, stirring gently. Remove from the heat.

5. Spoon the quinoa onto a platter. Top with the onion mixture. Sprinkle with the feta and parsley.

Exchanges / Choices
1 Starch, 3 Vegetable, 1 Lean Meat

Calories	200	**Sodium**	430 mg
Calories from Fat	20	**Potassium**	540 mg
Total Fat	**2 g**	**Total Carbohydrate**	**34 g**
Saturated Fat	0 g	Dietary Fiber	9 g
Trans Fat	0 g	Sugars	8 g
Polyunsaturated Fat	1 g	**Protein**	**12 g**
Monounsaturated Fat	0.5 g	**Phosphorus**	**350 mg**
Cholesterol	**5 mg**		

STIR-FRY VEGETABLES AND BROWN RICE

Serves 4 / Serving Size: 1 1/4 cups tofu mixture and 1/2 cup rice

A frozen vegetable blend combines with asparagus and tofu, then takes on an Asian flair when flavored with a savory sauce of soy, green onions, garlic, and crushed red pepper flakes. The toothsome mélange rests on a bed of nutty brown rice. If you're in a hurry, use 2 cups frozen brown rice.

1/2 cup uncooked brown rice

2 teaspoons canola or corn oil

1/4 cup plus 2 tablespoons sliced green onions (green part only), divided use

1 teaspoon minced peeled gingerroot

1 medium garlic clove, minced

1/4 teaspoon crushed red pepper flakes

4 ounces asparagus, trimmed and cut diagonally into 1-inch pieces

16 ounces frozen unseasoned broccoli stir-fry vegetables or a combination of your choice

8 ounces light firm tofu, drained, patted dry, and cut into 1/2-inch cubes

1/3 cup fat-free, low-sodium vegetable broth

1 tablespoon soy sauce (lowest sodium available)

1 tablespoon plain rice vinegar or white wine vinegar

2 teaspoons cornstarch

3 tablespoons water

1. Prepare the rice using the package directions, omitting the salt and margarine. Set aside.

2. About 10 minutes before the rice is ready, in a large nonstick skillet or wok, heat the oil over medium heat, swirling to coat the bottom. Cook 1/4 cup green onions, the gingerroot, garlic, and red pepper flakes for 1 minute, stirring occasionally.

3. Increase the heat to medium high. Add the asparagus. Cook for 1 minute, stirring frequently.

4. Stir in the stir-fry vegetables and tofu. Cook for 4–6 minutes, or until the vegetables are tender-crisp, stirring constantly.

5. Stir in the broth, soy sauce, and vinegar. Cook for 1 minute, stirring occasionally.

6. Put the cornstarch in a cup. Add the water, stirring to dissolve. Stir into the vegetable mixture. Cook for 1 minute, or until the mixture is thickened, stirring frequently.

7. Spoon the rice onto a platter. Top with the asparagus mixture. Sprinkle with the remaining 2 tablespoons green onions.

Exchanges / Choices
1 Starch, 3 Vegetable, 1 Lean Meat

Calories	190	Sodium	240 mg
Calories from Fat	35	Potassium	490 mg
Total Fat	**4 g**	**Total Carbohydrate**	**30 g**
Saturated Fat	0 g	Dietary Fiber	4 g
Trans Fat	0 g	Sugars	6 g
Polyunsaturated Fat	1 g	**Protein**	**9 g**
Monounsaturated Fat	2 g	**Phosphorus**	**180 mg**
Cholesterol	**0 mg**		

MEXICAN YELLOW RICE AND BLACK BEANS

Serves 4 / Serving Size: 1 1/2 cups

So much color in one simple dish! Black beans and red bell peppers nest on a cushion of turmeric-tinted rice, with orange cheddar and dark green cilantro sprinkled over all. With smoky cumin and a dash of heat from the red pepper flakes and Anaheim pepper, the flavors are as vivid as the hues.

3/4 cup uncooked brown rice

1/2 teaspoon ground turmeric

Olive oil cooking spray

1 large onion, chopped

1 large Anaheim pepper, seeds and ribs discarded, chopped (about 5 ounces), or 1 medium green bell pepper, chopped

1 medium red bell pepper, chopped

1/8 teaspoon crushed red pepper flakes

1 (15.5-ounce) can no-salt-added black beans, rinsed and drained

1/2 teaspoon ground cumin

1/4 teaspoon salt

1 tablespoon olive oil

2 ounces fat-free cheddar cheese, shredded

1/4 cup chopped fresh cilantro

2 medium limes, each cut into 4 wedges

1. Prepare the rice using the package directions, adding the turmeric and omitting the salt and margarine. Set aside.

2. Meanwhile, lightly spray a large skillet with cooking spray. Heat over medium-high heat. Remove from the heat. Put the onion, Anaheim pepper, bell pepper, and red pepper flakes in the skillet. Lightly spray with cooking spray. Cook for 4 minutes, or until the vegetables are beginning to lightly brown on the edges, stirring frequently. Remove from the heat.

3. Gently stir in the beans, cumin, and salt. Let stand, covered, for 5 minutes. Gently stir in the oil.

4. Spoon the rice onto a platter. Top with the bean mixture. Sprinkle with the cheddar and cilantro. Serve with the lime wedges.

Cook's Tip: Don't underestimate the power of fresh lime juice. It gives a lot of zing to this dish, which can also be used to serve 12 as a side dish.

Exchanges / Choices
3 Starch, 1 Vegetable, 1 Lean Meat

Calories	340	Sodium	340 mg
Calories from Fat	50	Potassium	770 mg
Total Fat	6 g	Total Carbohydrate	61 g
Saturated Fat	1 g	Dietary Fiber	10 g
Trans Fat	0 g	Sugars	10 g
Polyunsaturated Fat	1 g	Protein	14 g
Monounsaturated Fat	3 g	Phosphorus	375 mg
Cholesterol	<5 mg		

RED BEANS AND BROWN RICE

Serves 4 / Serving Size: 1 1/2 cups

In Louisiana, this down-home food was customarily prepared on wash day, an all-day event before washing machines and dryers. That meant wash day was a good time to set a slow-cooking pot of dried beans on the stove to simmer. By the time the clothes were done, the beans were, too. This recipe calls for canned beans, so you can enjoy it anytime, wash day or not!

1 1/2 teaspoons olive oil

1 medium onion, chopped

1 medium green bell pepper, chopped

1 medium red bell pepper, chopped

1/2 medium carrot, finely chopped

2 medium garlic cloves, minced

1/2 cup uncooked brown rice

1 teaspoon dried thyme, crumbled

1 teaspoon ground cumin

1/4 teaspoon crushed red pepper flakes

1/4 teaspoon salt

1 (14.5-ounce) can no-salt-added diced tomatoes, undrained

1 (8-ounce) can no-salt-added tomato sauce

1 cup water

1 (15.5-ounce) can no-salt-added kidney beans, rinsed and drained

1. In a large skillet, heat the oil over medium-high heat, swirling to coat the bottom. Cook the onion, bell peppers, carrot, and garlic for 3–4 minutes, or until the onion is soft, stirring occasionally.

2. Stir in the rice, thyme, cumin, red pepper flakes, and salt. Cook for 1 minute, stirring to coat the rice.

3. Stir in the tomatoes with liquid, tomato sauce, and water. Increase the heat to high and bring to a boil. Reduce the heat and simmer, covered, for 50 minutes, or until the rice is almost tender.

4. Stir in the beans. Cook for 10–15 minutes, or until the rice is tender and most of the liquid is absorbed.

Exchanges / Choices	
2 Starch, 3 Vegetable	

Calories	260	**Sodium**	150 mg
Calories from Fat	30	**Potassium**	1030 mg
Total Fat	**3 g**	**Total Carbohydrate**	**49 g**
Saturated Fat	0.5 g	Dietary Fiber	14 g
Trans Fat	0 g	Sugars	10 g
Polyunsaturated Fat	0.5 g	**Protein**	**11 g**
Monounsaturated Fat	1.5 g	**Phosphorus**	260 mg
Cholesterol	**0 mg**		

CREOLE RED BEAN RATATOUILLE

Serves 4 / Serving Size: 1 cup ratatouille and 1/2 cup pasta

Ratatouille is a classic vegetable dish from the Provence region of France. Our Creole-inspired version includes red kidney beans and whole-grain penne to add protein and fiber. Try it with Farmers' Market Veggie Salad (page 29). *(See photo insert.)*

4 ounces dried whole-grain penne

1 tablespoon olive oil (extra virgin preferred), divided use

1 medium onion, chopped

1 medium green bell pepper, chopped

2 medium garlic cloves, minced

4 medium tomatoes, chopped

1 cup frozen cut okra

1/2 (15.5-ounce) can no-salt-added kidney beans, rinsed and drained

3 medium dried bay leaves

1 teaspoon dried oregano, crumbled

1/2 teaspoon dried thyme, crumbled

1/8–1/4 teaspoon crushed red pepper flakes

1/4 cup chopped fresh parsley

1/2 teaspoon salt

2 ounces shredded low-fat mozzarella cheese

2 tablespoons shredded or grated Parmesan cheese

1. Prepare the pasta using the package directions, omitting the salt. Drain well in a colander. Set aside.

2. Meanwhile, in a large nonstick skillet, heat 1 teaspoon oil over medium-high heat, swirling to coat the bottom. Cook the onion and bell pepper for 3–4 minutes, or until soft, stirring frequently. Stir in the garlic. Cook for 10 seconds, stirring constantly. Stir in the tomatoes, okra, beans, bay leaves, oregano, thyme, and red pepper flakes. Bring to a simmer. Reduce the heat and simmer, covered, for 20 minutes, or until the okra is tender. Remove from the heat. Discard the bay leaves.

3. Stir the parsley, salt, and the remaining 2 teaspoons oil into the ratatouille. Serve over the pasta. Sprinkle with the mozzarella and Parmesan.

Exchanges / Choices
2 Starch, 2 Vegetable, 1 Medium-Fat Meat

Calories	280	Sodium	370 mg
Calories from Fat	60	Potassium	740 mg
Total Fat	**7 g**	**Total Carbohydrate**	**41 g**
Saturated Fat	2 g	Dietary Fiber	10 g
Trans Fat	0 g	Sugars	7 g
Polyunsaturated Fat	1 g	**Protein**	**15 g**
Monounsaturated Fat	3 g	**Phosphorus**	**275 mg**
Cholesterol	**5 mg**		

BEAN AND CHEESE TOSTADAS

Serves 4 / Serving Size: 1 tostada

A combination of giant nachos and tossed salad, these yummy tostadas require knives and forks. Creamy Frozen Fruit Wedges (page 175) provide a sweet, cooling finish to the meal.

1 (15.5-ounce) can no-salt-added pinto beans, rinsed and drained

1/4 cup water

2 teaspoons chili powder

1 teaspoon ground cumin

1 medium garlic clove, minced

1/4 teaspoon red hot-pepper sauce

4 (6-inch) corn tortillas

1/2 cup shredded low-fat sharp cheddar cheese

2 cups shredded romaine

4 ounces grape tomatoes or cherry tomatoes, quartered

1/3 cup finely chopped red onion

1/4 cup chopped fresh cilantro

1 tablespoon fresh lime juice

2 teaspoons olive oil

1/4 teaspoon salt

1. Preheat the oven to 350°F.

2. In a food processor or blender, process the beans, water, chili powder, cumin, garlic, and hot-pepper sauce until smooth.

3. Put the tortillas on a baking sheet. Spread the bean mixture on the tortillas. Sprinkle with the cheddar.

4. Bake for 10 minutes, or until the cheddar has melted and the bean mixture is hot.

5. Meanwhile, in a medium bowl, gently toss together the remaining ingredients.

6. Top the tortillas with the romaine mixture. Serve immediately.

Exchanges / Choices
2 Starch, 1 Lean Meat

Calories	210	**Sodium**	260 mg
Calories from Fat	40	**Potassium**	610 mg
Total Fat	4.5 g	**Total Carbohydrate**	31 g
Saturated Fat	1 g	Dietary Fiber	12 g
Trans Fat	0 g	Sugars	2 g
Polyunsaturated Fat	0.5 g	**Protein**	13 g
Monounsaturated Fat	2.5 g	**Phosphorus**	305 mg
Cholesterol	<5 mg		

VEGETARIAN TACOS

Serves 4 / Serving Size: 2 tacos

These tacos don't require any cooking, which makes it easy for you to put together a quick meal and be on your way. The bean mixture is also delicious when topping a salad of mixed greens.

1 cup canned no-salt-added kidney beans, rinsed and drained

1/2 cup frozen whole-kernel corn, thawed

1 small Italian plum (Roma) tomato, diced

1/2 small avocado, diced

2 tablespoons chopped fresh cilantro

1 tablespoon fresh lemon juice

1/2 teaspoon chili powder

8 (6-inch) corn tortillas

1/2 cup shredded romaine

1/2 cup shredded low-fat cheddar cheese

1/2 cup salsa (lowest sodium available)

1/4 cup chopped green onions

Exchanges / Choices

2 Starch, 2 Vegetable, 1 Lean Meat

Calories	250	**Sodium**	370 mg
Calories from Fat	45	**Potassium**	670 mg
Total Fat	5 g	**Total Carbohydrate**	41 g
Saturated Fat	1.5 g	Dietary Fiber	11 g
Trans Fat	0 g	Sugars	4 g
Polyunsaturated Fat	1 g	**Protein**	13 g
Monounsaturated Fat	2.5 g	**Phosphorus**	355 mg
Cholesterol	<5 mg		

1. In a small bowl, gently stir together the beans, corn, tomato, avocado, cilantro, lemon juice, and chili powder.

2. Spoon 1/4 cup bean mixture down the center of each tortilla. Top with the romaine, cheddar, salsa, and green onions. Fold the sides of the tortillas over the filling.

VEGETABLE CHILI WITH MIXED BEANS

Serves 4 / Serving Size: 2 cups

Cumin, paprika, green chiles, and chili powder season this meatless version of a popular standby that includes a variety of veggies and two types of beans. Try it over brown rice, barley, or even baked sweet potato halves to soak up every drop.

2 teaspoons canola or corn oil

1 large onion, chopped

1 medium bell pepper (any color), chopped

1 medium rib of celery, chopped

1 medium carrot, chopped

4 ounces button or brown (cremini) mushrooms, chopped

1/4 ounce dried oyster or porcini mushrooms, chopped

3 medium garlic cloves, minced

1/4 cup canned chopped green chiles, drained

1 teaspoon chili powder

1/2 teaspoon ground cumin

1/2 teaspoon paprika

1 (15.5-ounce) can no-salt-added kidney beans, rinsed and drained

1 (15.5-ounce) can no-salt-added cannellini beans, rinsed and drained

1 (14.5-ounce) can no-salt-added diced tomatoes, undrained

1 1/2 cups fat-free, low-sodium vegetable broth or water

1 (8-ounce) can no-salt-added tomato sauce

3 tablespoons chopped fresh cilantro

1. In a large nonstick saucepan, heat the oil over medium heat, swirling to coat the bottom. Cook the onion, bell pepper, celery, and carrot for 8–10 minutes, or until the carrot is tender, stirring frequently. Increase the heat to medium high.

2. Stir in the fresh mushrooms, dried mushrooms, and garlic. Cook for 2–4 minutes, or until the fresh mushrooms begin to soften.

3. Stir in the green chiles, chili powder, cumin, and paprika. Cook for 1 minute.

4. Stir in the remaining ingredients except the cilantro. Bring to a boil. Reduce the heat and simmer, partially covered, for 30 minutes.

5. Stir in the cilantro. Cook for 1 minute.

Exchanges / Choices	
2 1/2 Starch, 4 Vegetable, 1 Lean Meat	

Calories	340	Sodium	100 mg
Calories from Fat	30	Potassium	1400 mg
Total Fat	**3.5 g**	**Total Carbohydrate**	**60 g**
Saturated Fat	0.5 g	Dietary Fiber	21 g
Trans Fat	0 g	Sugars	10 g
Polyunsaturated Fat	1 g	**Protein**	**20 g**
Monounsaturated Fat	1.5 g	**Phosphorus**	**405 mg**
Cholesterol	**0 mg**		

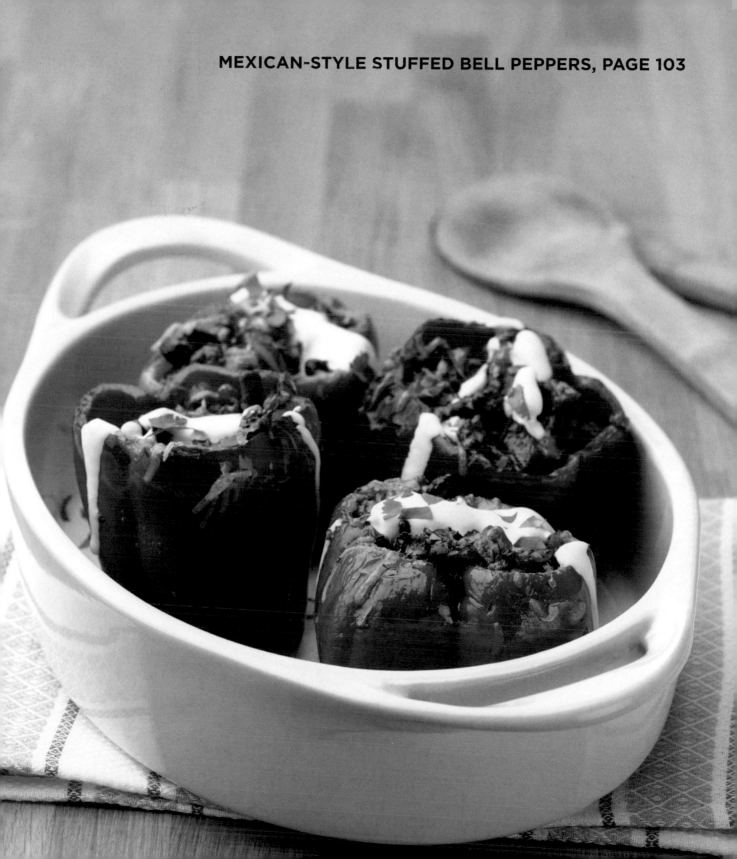

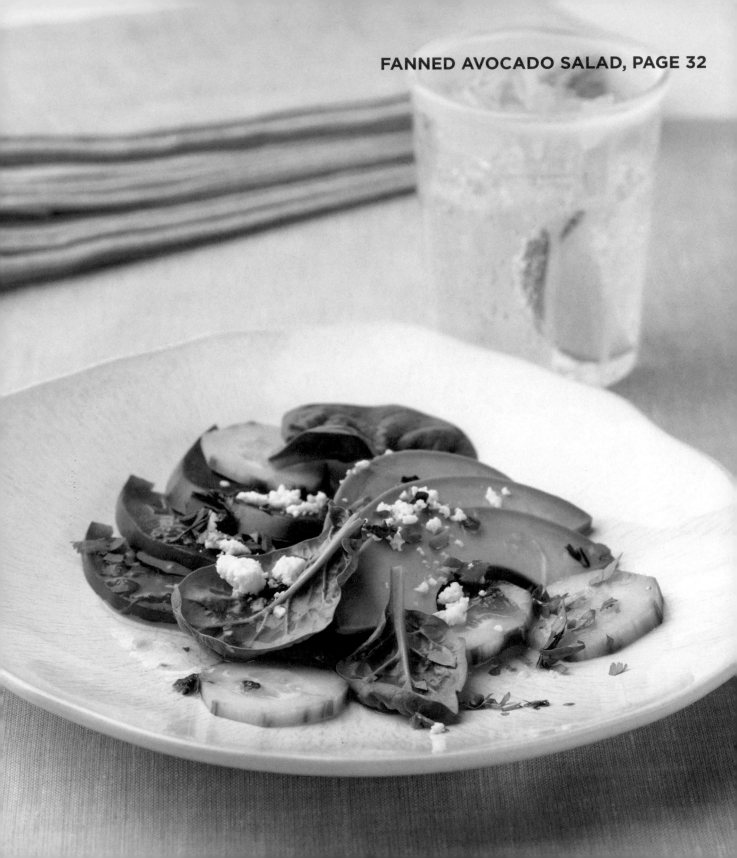

FANNED AVOCADO SALAD, PAGE 32

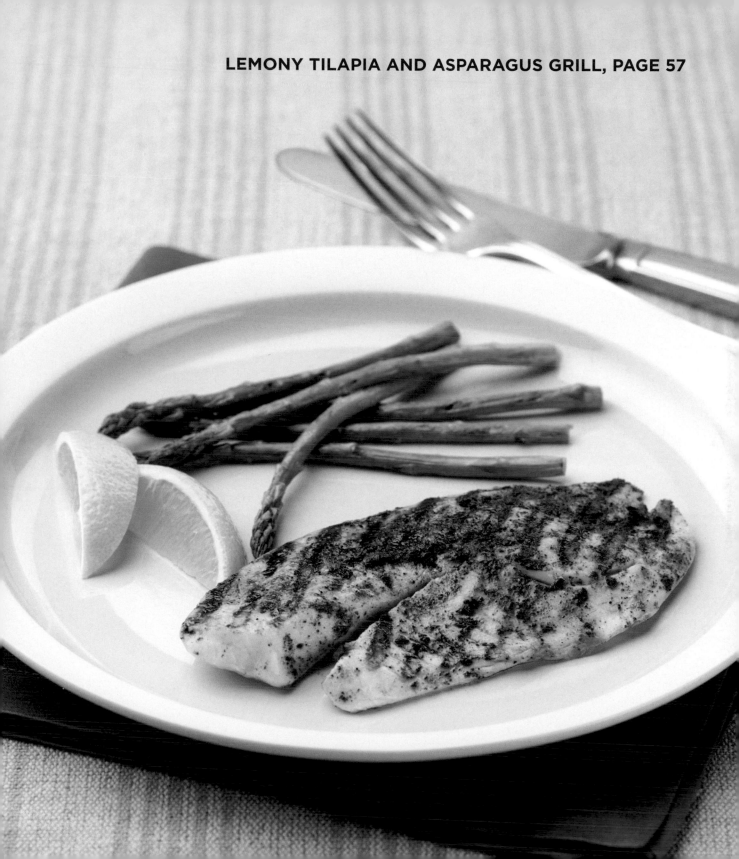

LEMONY TILAPIA AND ASPARAGUS GRILL, PAGE 57

OVEN-FRIED HADDOCK SANDWICH, PAGE 48

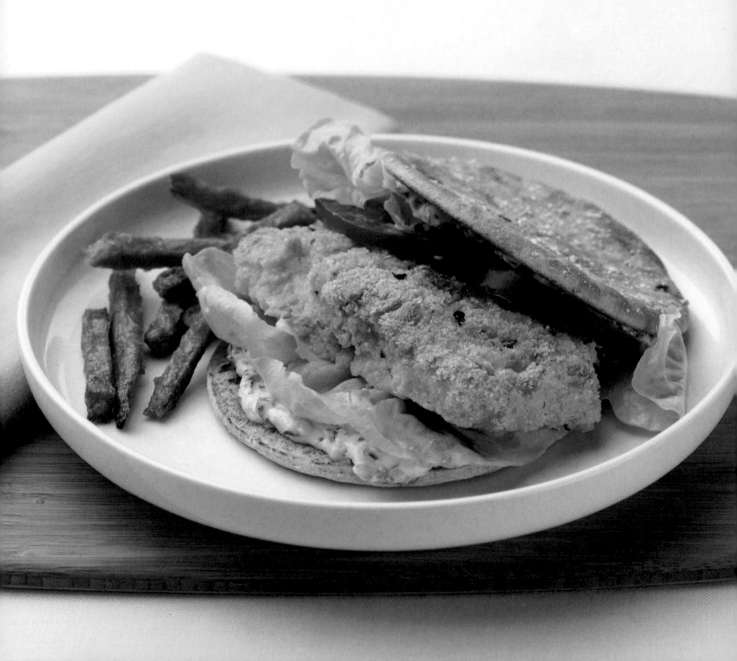

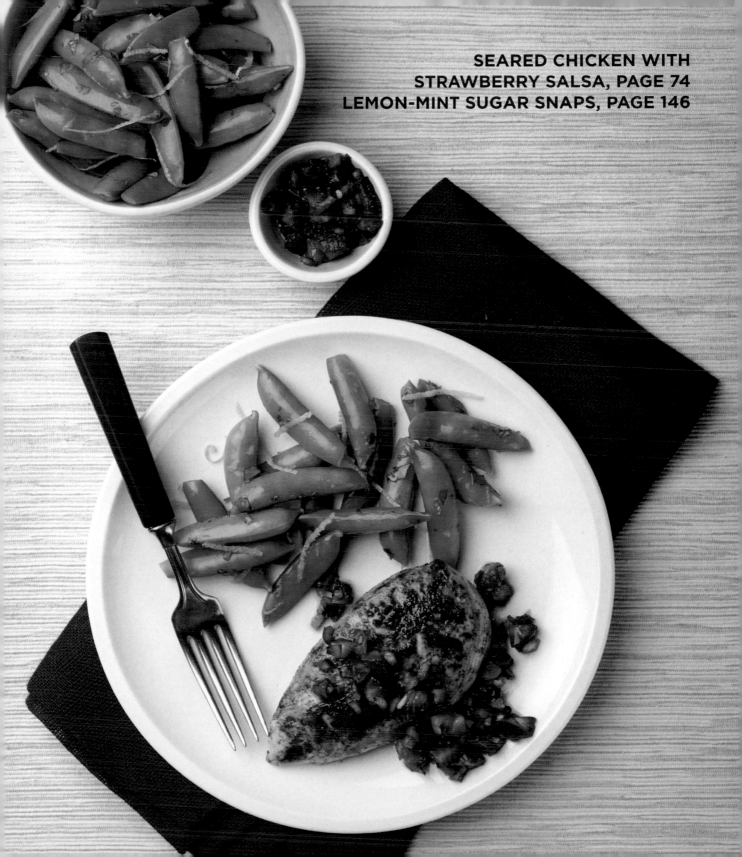

SEARED CHICKEN WITH STRAWBERRY SALSA, PAGE 74
LEMON-MINT SUGAR SNAPS, PAGE 146

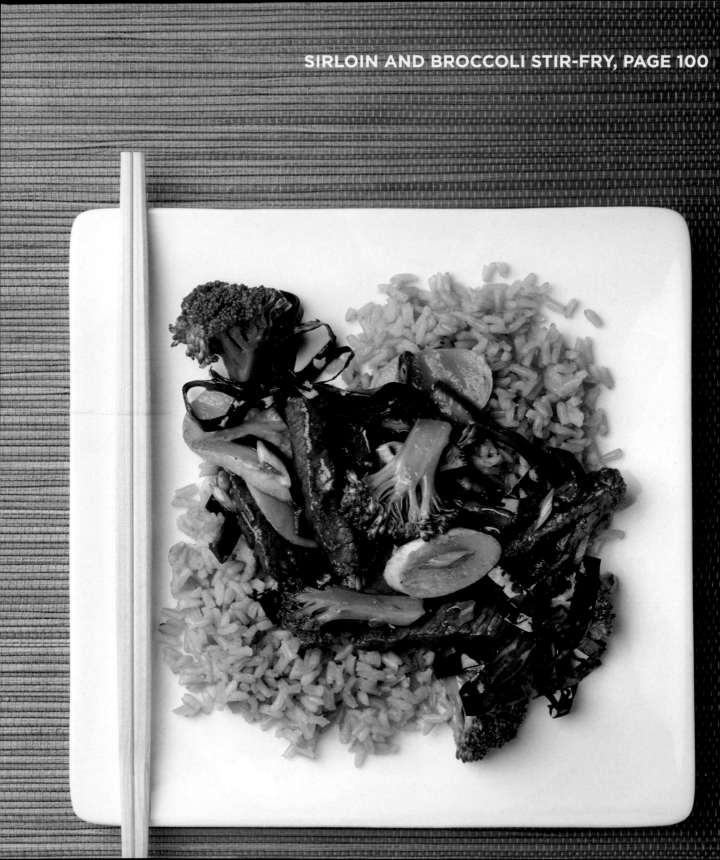

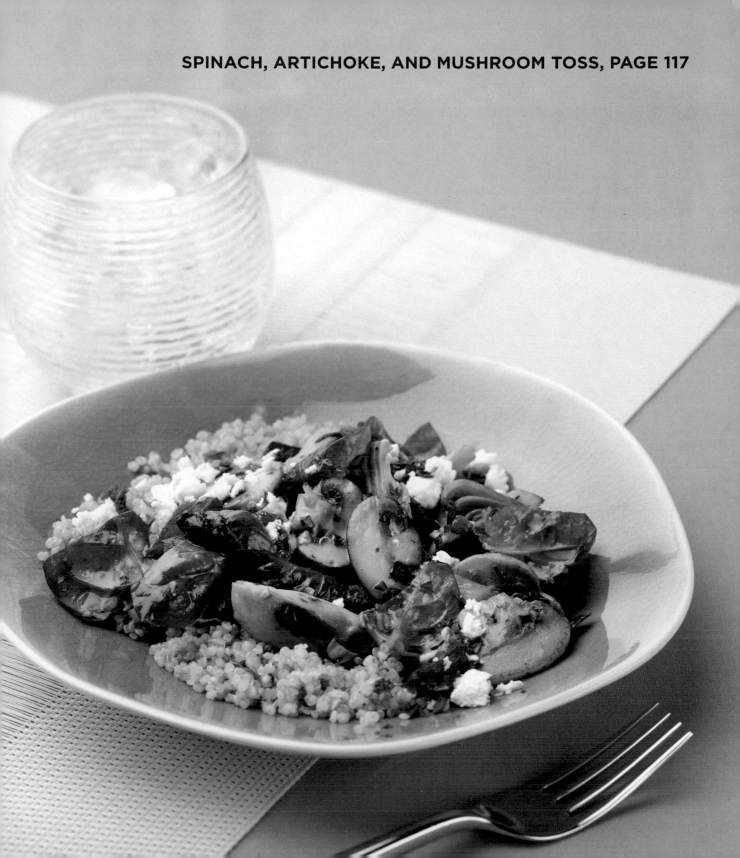

SPINACH, ARTICHOKE, AND MUSHROOM TOSS, PAGE 117

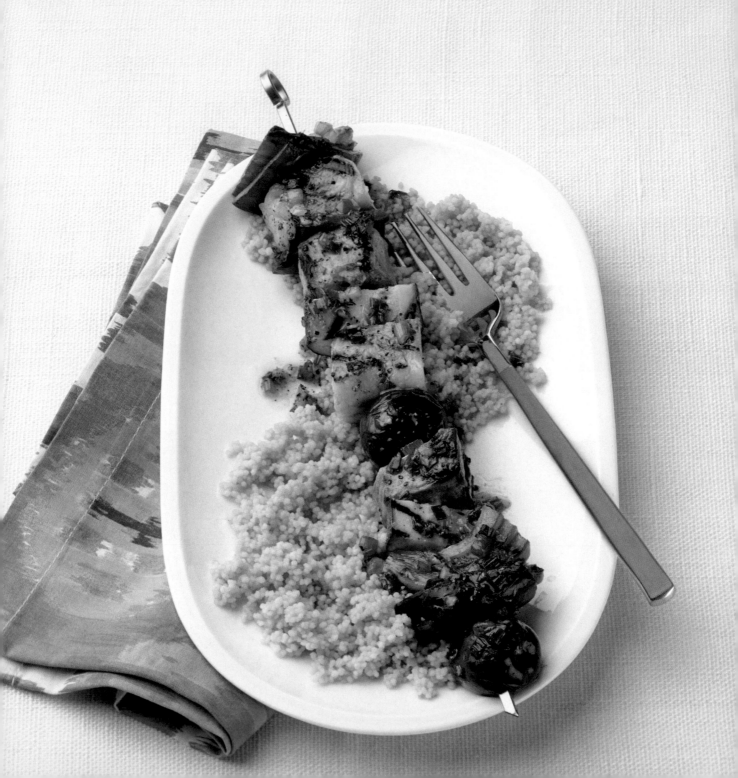

CHEESY WHITE BEAN AND FARRO CASSEROLE

Serves 4 / Serving Size: 1 1/2 cups

Rich-tasting, creamy melted cheddar cheese covers a hearty casserole featuring nutty cannellini beans and farro, an ancient whole grain popular in Italy. If you can't find it, you can use brown rice instead.

1 cup uncooked pearled farro

Cooking spray

1 (15.5-ounce) can no-salt-added cannellini beans, rinsed and drained

3/4 cup finely chopped green onions

4 ounces canned chopped green chiles, drained

3 tablespoons fresh lime juice

1 tablespoon ground cumin

1/8–1/4 teaspoon cayenne

1/8 teaspoon salt

1 cup shredded low-fat cheddar cheese

Exchanges / Choices
4 1/2 Carbohydrate, 1 Lean Meat

Calories	400	Sodium	410 mg
Calories from Fat	30	Potassium	730 mg
Total Fat	**3.5 g**	**Total Carbohydrate**	**66 g**
Saturated Fat	1.5 g	Dietary Fiber	11 g
Trans Fat	0 g	Sugars	2 g
Polyunsaturated Fat	0.5 g	**Protein**	**27 g**
Monounsaturated Fat	1 g	**Phosphorus**	**300 mg**
Cholesterol	**5 mg**		

1. Prepare the farro using the package directions, omitting the salt. Fluff with a fork.

2. Meanwhile, preheat the oven to 400°F.

3. Lightly spray an 11 x 7 x 2-inch glass baking dish with cooking spray. In the baking dish, stir together the farro, beans, green onions, green chiles, lime juice, cumin, cayenne, and salt. Spread the mixture in the baking dish. Sprinkle with the cheddar.

4. Bake for 20 minutes, or until the cheddar has melted and the casserole is warmed through.

LENTILS WITH BROWN RICE AND MUSHROOMS

Serves 4 / Serving Size: 1 1/2 cups

This **vegetarian entrée provides an appealing combination** of flavors and textures, with bright notes of orange contrasting with the earthiness of lentils and mushrooms and the smokiness of ground cumin. Serve it with Cantaloupe Wedges with Ginger-Citrus Sauce (page 33) for a burst of color and refreshment.

3 cups fat-free, low-sodium vegetable broth or water

3/4 cup dried green or brown lentils, sorted for stones and shriveled lentils, rinsed, and drained

1/2 cup uncooked brown rice

2 teaspoons olive oil

1 large onion, chopped

2 cups chopped mushrooms, such as button, brown (cremini), portobello, or shiitake (stems discarded)

2 medium garlic cloves, minced

1 teaspoon ground cumin

1 teaspoon grated orange zest

3 tablespoons fresh orange juice

1/4 teaspoon crushed red pepper flakes

1 tablespoon soy sauce (lowest sodium available)

3 tablespoons minced fresh cilantro or parsley

1. In a medium saucepan, bring the broth to a boil over high heat. Stir in the lentils and return to a boil. Reduce the heat and simmer, covered, for 10 minutes.

2. Stir in the rice. Simmer, covered, for 25–30 minutes, or until the lentils and rice are tender and almost all the liquid is absorbed.

3. Meanwhile, in a medium nonstick skillet, heat the oil over medium-low heat, swirling to coat the bottom. Cook the onion, mushrooms, and garlic for 10–12 minutes, or until the onion is very soft and browned, stirring occasionally.

4. Stir in the cumin, orange zest, and red pepper flakes. Cook for 1 minute, stirring frequently.

5. Stir in the orange juice and soy sauce. Cook for 1 minute.

6. Stir the onion mixture and cilantro into the lentil mixture. Cook for 1 minute, or until hot.

Exchanges / Choices
3 Starch, 1 Vegetable

Calories	280	**Sodium**	260 mg
Calories from Fat	35	**Potassium**	720 mg
Total Fat	**4 g**	**Total Carbohydrate**	**49 g**
Saturated Fat	0.5 g	Dietary Fiber	14 g
Trans Fat	0 g	Sugars	6 g
Polyunsaturated Fat	0.5 g	**Protein**	**13 g**
Monounsaturated Fat	2 g	**Phosphorus**	**290 mg**
Cholesterol	**0 mg**		

LENTIL STEW WITH VEGETARIAN SAUSAGE

Serves 4 / Serving Size: 1 1/2 cups

A bowl of this satisfying stew, full of vegetables, lentils, and veggie sausage, might very well become a new family favorite. It pairs beautifully with Salad Greens with Mixed-Herb Vinaigrette (page 25).

2 teaspoons olive oil

1 cup chopped onion

1 cup sliced baby carrots or 2 medium carrots, sliced crosswise

1 small sweet potato, chopped

1 medium rib of celery, sliced crosswise

1/2 medium green bell pepper, chopped

2 medium garlic cloves, minced

1/2 cup dried lentils, sorted for stones and shriveled lentils, rinsed, and drained

1 tablespoon chopped fresh thyme or 1 teaspoon dried thyme, crumbled

1 teaspoon ground cumin

1/2 teaspoon dry mustard

3 cups fat-free, low-sodium vegetable broth or water

1 (14.5-ounce) can no-salt-added diced tomatoes, undrained

2/3 cup water

2 medium dried bay leaves

1/4 teaspoon pepper

4 ounces vegetarian sausage or vegetarian hot dogs (lowest sodium available), sliced

2 tablespoons red wine vinegar

1. In a large saucepan, heat the oil over medium heat, swirling to coat the bottom. Cook the onion for 3–4 minutes, or until tender, stirring frequently.

2. Stir in the carrots, sweet potato, celery, bell pepper, and garlic. Cook for 5 minutes, stirring frequently.

3. Stir in the lentils, thyme, cumin, and mustard. Cook for 1 minute, stirring to coat the lentils.

4. Increase the heat to medium high. Stir in the broth, tomatoes with liquid, water, bay leaves, and pepper. Bring to a boil. Skim off any foam. Reduce the heat and simmer, covered, for 25 minutes. The lentils will still be firm.

5. Stir in the sausage and vinegar. Cook for 5–7 minutes, or until the lentils are tender. Discard the bay leaves.

Cook's Tip: The cooking time for lentils varies from about 25 minutes for red lentils to about 45 minutes for most other varieties.

Exchanges / Choices

1 1/2 Starch, 3 Vegetable

Calories	260	**Sodium**	420 mg
Calories from Fat	50	**Potassium**	1020 mg
Total Fat	**6 g**	**Total Carbohydrate**	**40 g**
Saturated Fat	1 g	Dietary Fiber	13 g
Trans Fat	0 g	Sugars	10 g
Polyunsaturated Fat	1.5 g	**Protein**	**14 g**
Monounsaturated Fat	3.5 g	**Phosphorus**	**240 mg**
Cholesterol	**0 mg**		

CRUSTLESS ASPARAGUS AND TOMATO QUICHE

Serves 4 / Serving Size: 1/4 quiche

With no crust needed, this quiche is so simple to prepare. Sweet grape tomatoes help create a nice balance of flavors and textures and add a striking color contrast with the bright green asparagus. Try it with a mixed-greens salad or a cup of Tomato Basil Bisque (page 13).

Cooking spray

1 teaspoon canola or corn oil

10 ounces asparagus, trimmed and cut diagonally into 2-inch pieces

4 medium green onions, chopped

12 grape or cherry tomatoes, halved

1 cup fat-free milk or fat-free evaporated milk

4 large egg whites

2 large eggs

2 teaspoons Dijon mustard (lowest sodium available)

1 1/2 teaspoons chopped fresh thyme or 1/2 teaspoon dried thyme, crumbled

1/4 teaspoon pepper

1/2 cup shredded or grated low-fat cheddar or Colby cheese

1. Preheat the oven to 350°F. Lightly spray a 9-inch glass pie pan with cooking spray.

2. In a medium nonstick skillet, heat the oil over medium heat, swirling to coat the bottom. Cook the asparagus and green onions for 4–5 minutes, or until soft. Arrange the asparagus mixture and the tomatoes with the cut side down in the pie pan.

3. In a medium bowl, whisk together the remaining ingredients except the cheddar. Pour the mixture over the vegetables. Sprinkle with the cheddar.

4. Bake for 30–35 minutes, or until a knife inserted in the center comes out clean. Let the quiche cool for about 10 minutes before slicing.

Exchanges / Choices
2 Vegetable, 2 Lean Meat

Calories	150	**Sodium**	280 mg
Calories from Fat	45	**Potassium**	500 mg
Total Fat	**5 g**	**Total Carbohydrate**	**10 g**
Saturated Fat	1.5 g	Dietary Fiber	3 g
Trans Fat	0 g	Sugars	7 g
Polyunsaturated Fat	1 g	**Protein**	**15 g**
Monounsaturated Fat	2 g	**Phosphorus**	250 mg
Cholesterol	**100 mg**		

SKILLET-ROASTED VEGGIE SCRAMBLE

Serves 4 / Serving Size: 1 tortilla stack

After you've tried this dish for dinner, you'll want to have it for breakfast and brunch as well. Serve it with a mixture of fresh seasonal fruit for a light, refreshing meal at any time of day.

Cooking spray

1 large onion, chopped

1 medium bell pepper (any color), chopped

1 medium yellow summer squash, diced

4 ounces sliced mushrooms, such as button, brown (cremini), portobello, or shiitake (stems discarded)

1/2 teaspoon dried oregano, crumbled

1/4 cup water

1/8 teaspoon salt

1/8 teaspoon cayenne

4 large egg whites

2 large eggs

3 tablespoons fat-free milk

4 (6-inch) corn tortillas

3/4 cup shredded low-fat sharp cheddar cheese

1. Lightly spray a large skillet with cooking spray. Heat over medium-high heat. Cook the onion, bell pepper, and squash for 3 minutes, or until the onion is soft, stirring occasionally.

2. Stir in the mushrooms and oregano. Cook for 6 minutes, or until the mushrooms are just beginning to lightly brown on the edges, stirring constantly. Transfer the onion mixture to a medium bowl.

3. Pour the water into the skillet, scraping to dislodge any browned bits. Stir in the onion mixture, salt, and cayenne. Remove from the heat.

4. In a small bowl, whisk together the egg whites, eggs, and milk.

5. Lightly spray a separate large skillet with cooking spray. Heat over medium heat. Pour the egg mixture into the skillet, swirling to coat the bottom. Cook for 30 seconds, or until beginning to set. Using a spatula, carefully lift the cooked edge and tilt the skillet so the uncooked portion flows under the edge. Cook for 1–2 minutes, or until no runniness remains, repeating the lift-and-tilt procedure once or twice at other places along the edge if needed.

6. Put the tortillas on plates. Spoon the egg mixture onto each tortilla. Top with the onion mixture. Sprinkle with the cheddar.

Cook's Tip: If you want to slightly melt the cheddar topping, put the tortillas on a broiler rack instead of on plates. Assemble as directed, then broil the tortilla stacks about 6–8 inches from the heat for about 1 minute.

Exchanges / Choices
1 Carbohydrate, 2 Lean Meat

Calories	170	Sodium	310 mg
Calories from Fat	45	Potassium	430 mg
Total Fat	**5 g**	**Total Carbohydrate**	**16 g**
Saturated Fat	2 g	Dietary Fiber	3 g
Trans Fat	0 g	Sugars	3 g
Polyunsaturated Fat	1 g	**Protein**	**16 g**
Monounsaturated Fat	2 g	**Phosphorus**	**310 mg**
Cholesterol	**100 mg**		

ITALIAN EGGPLANT

Serves 4 / Serving Size: 1 eggplant stack

A slice of eggplant is the base for each serving of this rich-tasting mixture of vegetables, tomato sauce, and creamy cheese. Try it with a side of whole-grain pasta and Italian Skillet Spinach (page 143).

1 (1-pound) unpeeled eggplant, cut crosswise into 1/2-inch slices

Cooking spray

1 cup chopped zucchini

1 large onion, chopped

1 medium rib of celery, finely chopped

2 teaspoons dried oregano, crumbled

2 medium garlic cloves, minced

1/4 teaspoon crushed red pepper flakes

1/3 cup water

2 slices whole-wheat bread (lowest sodium available), processed into very fine crumbs

2 large egg whites

1/8 teaspoon salt

1/2 cup spaghetti sauce, such as tomato basil (lowest sodium available)

3/4 cup shredded low-fat mozzarella cheese

2 tablespoons shredded or grated Parmesan cheese

1. Preheat the oven to 350°F.

2. Select the 4 largest eggplant slices. Lightly spray both sides with cooking spray. Transfer them to a nonstick baking sheet. Set aside. Chop the remaining eggplant slices into 1/2-inch pieces.

3. Lightly spray a large skillet with cooking spray. Heat over medium-high heat. Remove from the heat. Put the chopped eggplant, zucchini, onion, celery, oregano, garlic, and red pepper flakes into the skillet. Lightly spray the vegetables with cooking spray. Cook for 8 minutes, or until the eggplant is tender, stirring frequently. Remove from the heat.

4. Stir in the water. Stir in the bread crumbs, egg whites, and salt. Spoon the chopped eggplant mixture onto each eggplant slice.

5. Bake for 25 minutes, or until the eggplant slices are tender. Top each with the spaghetti sauce. Sprinkle with the mozzarella. Bake for 5 minutes, or until the mozzarella has melted. Remove from the oven.

6. Sprinkle with the Parmesan. Let stand for 5 minutes before serving.

Exchanges / Choices
3 Vegetable, 1 1/2 Starch, 1 Lean Meat, 1 Fat

Calories	180	**Sodium**	290 mg
Calories from Fat	45	Potassium	570 mg
Total Fat	5 g	**Total Carbohydrate**	20 g
Saturated Fat	2 g	Dietary Fiber	6 g
Trans Fat	0 g	Sugars	7 g
Polyunsaturated Fat	0.5 g	**Protein**	13 g
Monounsaturated Fat	0.5 g	**Phosphorus**	200 mg
Cholesterol	10 mg		

| *Vegetables and Side Dishes* |

PECAN-ROASTED ASPARAGUS

Serves 4 / Serving Size: 5 asparagus spears

Roasting brings out the best of both the asparagus and the pecans in this simple dish, which is an elegant match for Mustard-Crusted Beef Tenderloin (page 90). Turn the oven down a notch and let the asparagus cook while the beef is resting, so they're both done at the same time.

1 pound asparagus spears (about 20 spears), trimmed, dried completely after rinsing

2 tablespoons finely chopped pecans

Cooking spray

1 tablespoon sugar

1 tablespoon balsamic vinegar

1/8 teaspoon salt

1. Preheat the oven to 425°F.

2. Arrange the asparagus in a single layer on a baking sheet. Sprinkle with the pecans. Lightly spray with cooking spray.

3. Roast for 10 minutes, or until the asparagus is tender-crisp and the pecans are browned.

4. Meanwhile, in a small bowl, whisk together the sugar, vinegar, and salt.

5. Remove the asparagus from the oven. Pour the sugar mixture over the asparagus. Stir gently.

Exchanges / Choices
2 Vegetable, 1/2 Fat

Calories	60	**Sodium**	55 mg
Calories from Fat	30	**Potassium**	250 mg
Total Fat	3 g	**Total Carbohydrate**	9 g
Saturated Fat	0 g	Dietary Fiber	3 g
Trans Fat	0 g	Sugars	6 g
Polyunsaturated Fat	1 g	**Protein**	3 g
Monounsaturated Fat	1.5 g	**Phosphorus**	70 mg
Cholesterol	0 mg		

TOASTED-ALMOND RICE AND PEAS

Serves 6 / Serving Size: 1/2 cup

Rice tossed with sweet green peas and crunchy almonds is a perfect foil for Asian fare or a simple roast chicken. The turmeric adds a distinctive bright yellow hue and an exotic fragrance to the rice.

1 cup uncooked brown rice

1/2 teaspoon ground turmeric

3 tablespoons sliced almonds, dry-roasted

3/4 cup frozen green peas, thawed

1/4 cup finely chopped green onions

1/4 teaspoon salt

1. Prepare the rice using the package directions, omitting the salt and margarine and adding the turmeric. Transfer to a large bowl.

2. Stir in the remaining ingredients.

Cook's Tip: Save some time by dry-roasting the nuts for several recipes at once. Let them cool completely. Store them in an airtight container at room temperature for up to two weeks or freeze for longer storage.

Exchanges / Choices
2 Starch

Calories	150	**Sodium**	85 mg
Calories from Fat	25	**Potassium**	140 mg
Total Fat	2.5 g	**Total Carbohydrate**	28 g
Saturated Fat	0 g	Dietary Fiber	3 g
Trans Fat	0 g	Sugars	1 g
Polyunsaturated Fat	0.5 g	**Protein**	4 g
Monounsaturated Fat	1 g	**Phosphorus**	115 mg
Cholesterol	0 mg		

ASIAN BROCCOLI WITH PECANS

Serves 4 / Serving Size: 1/2 cup

This sweet and nutty side dish is perfect for dressing up a simple entrée of chicken or pork, letting the broccoli get the attention it deserves. Two to try: Oven-Fried Sesame-Ginger Chicken (page 70) or Asian Barbecued Pork Tenderloin (page 106).

10 ounces broccoli florets

1 tablespoon sugar

1 tablespoon soy sauce (lowest sodium available)

1 tablespoon balsamic vinegar

1/2 teaspoon grated peeled gingerroot

1/8 teaspoon crushed red pepper flakes

2 tablespoons finely chopped pecans, dry-roasted

Exchanges / Choices
2 Vegetable, 1/2 Fat

Calories	60	**Sodium**	170 mg
Calories from Fat	25	**Potassium**	210 mg
Total Fat	**2.5 g**	**Total Carbohydrate**	**8 g**
Saturated Fat	0 g	Dietary Fiber	2 g
Trans Fat	0 g	Sugars	5 g
Polyunsaturated Fat	1 g	**Protein**	**1 g**
Monounsaturated Fat	1.5 g	**Phosphorus**	55 mg
Cholesterol	**0 mg**		

1. In a medium saucepan, steam the broccoli, covered, for 5 minutes, or until tender-crisp. Drain well.

2. Meanwhile, in a small bowl, whisk together the remaining ingredients except the pecans. (It isn't necessary for the sugar to dissolve completely.)

3. Arrange the broccoli on a platter. Spoon the sugar mixture over the broccoli. Sprinkle with the pecans.

EGGPLANT WITH ROASTED RED BELL PEPPER RELISH

Serves 6 / Serving Size: 2 slices eggplant and 1 heaping tablespoon relish

Roasted red bell pepper relish adds a burst of color and flavor atop thick slices of tender, lightly browned eggplant. Roasting the eggplant tames its slightly bitter flavor and highlights its natural richness. *(See photo insert.)*

Cooking spray

1 (1 1/2-pound) unpeeled eggplant, cut into 12 slices, each 1/2 inch

1 tablespoon olive oil, divided use

1/8 teaspoon salt

1/2 cup roasted red bell peppers, drained if bottled, chopped

1 tablespoon chopped fresh parsley or 1/4 teaspoon dried oregano, thyme, or basil, crumbled

1/2 teaspoon red wine vinegar

1 small garlic clove, minced

Pinch of pepper

Exchanges / Choices	
1 Vegetable, 1/2 Fat	

Calories	50	**Sodium**	200 mg
Calories from Fat	30	**Potassium**	280 mg
Total Fat	**3 g**	**Total Carbohydrate**	**7 g**
Saturated Fat	0.5 g	Dietary Fiber	3 g
Trans Fat	0 g	Sugars	4 g
Polyunsaturated Fat	0.5 g	**Protein**	**1 g**
Monounsaturated Fat	2 g	**Phosphorus**	30 mg
Cholesterol	**0 mg**		

1. Preheat the oven to 425°F. Lightly spray a large baking dish with cooking spray.

2. Lightly brush both sides of the eggplant slices with 2 teaspoons oil. Sprinkle the salt over the top of the slices. Arrange in a single layer in the baking dish.

3. Roast for 18–20 minutes, or until the eggplant is lightly browned on the bottom. Turn over. Roast for 8 minutes, or until browned on the bottom. Transfer the eggplant to plates.

4. Meanwhile, in a small bowl, stir together the remaining ingredients, including the remaining 1 teaspoon oil. Spoon over the eggplant.

GREEN BEANS WITH MUSHROOMS AND ONIONS

Serves 4 / Serving Size: 1/2 cup

Crisp, vibrant green beans and earthy mushrooms were meant for each other, as you'll experience when you taste this lightly flavored side dish. Try it with Mustard-Crusted Beef Tenderloin (page 90) or Turkey Marsala (page 84).

8 ounces green beans, trimmed

2 teaspoons olive oil

4 ounces sliced mushrooms, such as button, brown (cremini), portobello, or shiitake (stems discarded)

1/2 cup thinly sliced onion

1 medium garlic clove, minced

1/8 teaspoon salt

2 teaspoons fresh lemon juice

Pinch of pepper

Exchanges / Choices
2 Vegetable, 1/2 Fat

Calories	60	**Sodium**	60 mg
Calories from Fat	25	**Potassium**	300 mg
Total Fat	2.5 g	**Total Carbohydrate**	9 g
Saturated Fat	0.5 g	Dietary Fiber	2 g
Trans Fat	0 g	Sugars	4 g
Polyunsaturated Fat	0.5 g	**Protein**	2 g
Monounsaturated Fat	1.5 g	**Phosphorus**	70 mg
Cholesterol	0 mg		

1. Fill a medium saucepan three-fourths full with water. Bring to a boil, covered, over high heat. Cook the green beans, uncovered, for 5 minutes, or until tender-crisp. Drain well in a colander.

2. Meanwhile, in a medium nonstick skillet, heat the oil over medium-high heat, swirling to coat the bottom. Cook the mushrooms, onion, garlic, and salt for 5 minutes, or until the mushrooms are soft and lightly browned, stirring frequently. Stir in the lemon juice, pepper, and cooked green beans.

Cook's Tip: Covering the saucepan while bringing the water to a boil speeds up the process.

ROASTED GREEN BEANS DIJON

Serves 6 / Serving Size: 1/2 cup

These green beans are so easy to prepare that you'll want to serve them over and over again. Roasting enhances the vegetable's natural sweetness, which contrasts well with the mustard's trademark bite.

1 pound green beans, trimmed, dried completely after rinsing

Cooking spray

2 teaspoons olive oil

1/2 teaspoon Dijon mustard (lowest sodium available)

1/4 teaspoon salt

1/4 cup chopped fresh parsley

1. Preheat the oven to 425°F.

2. Put the green beans on a large baking sheet. Lightly spray them with cooking spray. Toss gently. Arrange the green beans in a single layer on the baking sheet. Lightly spray again.

3. Roast for 10 minutes, or until the green beans are tender.

4. Meanwhile, in a small bowl, whisk together the oil, mustard, and salt. Drizzle over the green beans. Stir gently. Sprinkle with the parsley.

Cook's Tip: Vegetables that are going to be roasted need to be completely dry. Any moisture will cause them to steam instead of roast and will keep them from browning.

Exchanges / Choices
1 Vegetable

Calories	40	Sodium	80 mg
Calories from Fat	20	Potassium	170 mg
Total Fat	2 g	Total Carbohydrate	6 g
Saturated Fat	0.5 g	Dietary Fiber	2 g
Trans Fat	0 g	Sugars	3 g
Polyunsaturated Fat	0.5 g	Protein	1 g
Monounsaturated Fat	1.5 g	Phosphorus	30 mg
Cholesterol	0 mg		

DOWN-HOME GREENS

Serves 4 / Serving Size: 3/4 cup

Pick your favorite greens—turnip, collard, or mustard—and don't forget the hot-pepper sauce! Try these with Onion-Smothered Pork Chops (page 109) or Chicken with Country Gravy (page 77) for a healthy meal, southern-style.

1 3/4 cups fat-free, low-sodium chicken broth

16 ounces frozen chopped turnip, collard, or mustard greens

1 teaspoon dried thyme, crumbled

1/2 teaspoon sugar

1/4 teaspoon crushed red pepper flakes

1/8 teaspoon red hot-pepper sauce, or to taste

Exchanges / Choices

2 Vegetable

Calories	60	Sodium	80 mg
Calories from Fat	10	Potassium	430 mg
Total Fat	1 g	**Total Carbohydrate**	10 g
Saturated Fat	0.5 g	Dietary Fiber	4 g
Trans Fat	0 g	Sugars	2 g
Polyunsaturated Fat	0 g	**Protein**	4 g
Monounsaturated Fat	0.5 g	Phosphorus	80 mg
Cholesterol	0 mg		

1. In a Dutch oven, bring the broth to a boil over high heat.

2. Stir in the remaining ingredients except the hot-pepper sauce. Return to a boil. Reduce the heat and simmer, covered, for 20 minutes, or until the greens are tender. Just before serving, sprinkle with the hot-pepper sauce.

MUSHROOMS MARINATED IN LIME AND SOY SAUCE

Serves 8 / Serving Size: 4 mushrooms

Whether you choose to broil these tender mushrooms or serve them raw, they are juiced up with fresh lime and brightened with a flash of chopped green parsley before serving. The mushrooms' meaty texture pairs particularly well with beef or pork.

32 small button mushrooms (about 1 pound)

1/4 cup soy sauce (lowest sodium available)

1/4 cup fresh lime juice

1 tablespoon olive oil

1/4 teaspoon crushed red pepper flakes

Cooking spray

2 medium limes, each cut into 4 wedges

1/4 cup chopped fresh parsley

Exchanges / Choices			
1 Vegetable			
Calories	30	**Sodium**	150 mg
Calories from Fat	10	**Potassium**	220 mg
Total Fat	**1 g**	**Total Carbohydrate**	**5 g**
Saturated Fat	0 g	Dietary Fiber	1 g
Trans Fat	0 g	Sugars	2 g
Polyunsaturated Fat	0 g	**Protein**	**2 g**
Monounsaturated Fat	1 g	**Phosphorus**	**60 mg**
Cholesterol	**0 mg**		

1. In a large shallow glass dish, stir together the mushrooms, soy sauce, lime juice, oil, and red pepper flakes. Cover and refrigerate for 8 hours, turning occasionally.

2. To serve chilled, drain the mushrooms, discarding the marinade.

3. To serve hot, preheat the broiler. Lightly spray a large baking sheet with cooking spray. Drain the mushrooms, discarding the marinade. Arrange the mushrooms in a single layer on the baking sheet with the stem sides down. Broil about 4–6 inches from the heat for 6 minutes, or until beginning to brown, stirring occasionally.

4. For both the raw and broiled mushrooms, just before serving, squeeze the lime over the mushrooms. Sprinkle with the parsley.

RED POTATOES PARMESAN

Serves 4 / Serving Size: 1/2 cup per serving

These steamed potatoes are coated with a blend of pungent Parmesan, creamy margarine, mild parsley, and delicate green onions. They're so quick and easy to prepare that they're perfect for busy weeknights when you need to get dinner ready in a rush.

12 ounces red potatoes, cut into 1/2-inch cubes

1/4 cup minced green onions

2 tablespoons chopped fresh parsley

2 tablespoons light tub margarine

1/8 teaspoon salt

2 tablespoons shredded or grated Parmesan cheese

1. Steam the potatoes, covered, for 8 minutes, or until tender when pierced with a fork. Drain well.

2. In a medium bowl, gently stir together the cooked potatoes and the remaining ingredients except the Parmesan.

3. Gently stir in the Parmesan.

Exchanges / Choices
1 Starch

Calories	100	**Sodium**	150 mg
Calories from Fat	35	**Potassium**	420 mg
Total Fat	**4 g**	**Total Carbohydrate**	**14 g**
Saturated Fat	1 g	Dietary Fiber	2 g
Trans Fat	0 g	Sugars	1 g
Polyunsaturated Fat	1 g	**Protein**	**3 g**
Monounsaturated Fat	1 g	**Phosphorus**	**75 mg**
Cholesterol	**<5 mg**		

SCALLOPED POTATOES

Serves 6 / Serving Size: 1/2 cup

Just slice russet potatoes, layer them with the goodness of sharp cheddar, sprinkle with savory chopped onion, and bake. Here's a dish that will warm your heart and make a tasty companion for roast chicken, fish, beef, or pork.

Cooking spray

1 pound russet potatoes, thinly sliced

1/4 cup finely chopped onion

2 tablespoons light tub margarine

1/4 teaspoon salt, divided use

1/8 teaspoon pepper

1/2 cup grated sharp low-fat cheddar or low-fat mozzarella cheese, divided use

1/2 cup fat-free milk, warmed

Exchanges / Choices			
1 Starch			
Calories	110	**Sodium**	170 mg
Calories from Fat	30	**Potassium**	370 mg
Total Fat	**3 g**	**Total Carbohydrate**	**16 g**
Saturated Fat	1 g	Dietary Fiber	1 g
Trans Fat	0 g	Sugars	2 g
Polyunsaturated Fat	1 g	**Protein**	**5 g**
Monounsaturated Fat	1 g	**Phosphorus**	120 mg
Cholesterol	**<5 mg**		

1. Preheat the oven to 425°F. Lightly spray a 9-inch glass pie pan with cooking spray.

2. Arrange half the potato slices in the pan. Sprinkle the onion on the potato. Using a teaspoon, dot with the margarine. Sprinkle 1/8 teaspoon salt, the pepper, and 1/4 cup cheddar over all. Top with the remaining potato slices. Pour the milk over all.

3. Bake for 30 minutes. Sprinkle with the remaining 1/4 cup cheddar and 1/8 teaspoon salt. Bake for 5 minutes, or until the cheddar has melted. Remove from the oven. Let stand for 5 minutes.

Cook's Tip: Russet potatoes will absorb the moisture in this dish, providing the desired starchiness.

RED PEPPER PILAF

Serves 6 / Serving Size: 1/2 cup

This golden pilaf dotted with red bell peppers and green parsley makes a colorful statement and its creamy, risottolike texture is undeniably appealing. The bell peppers and red pepper flakes together add a sweet heat.

1 1/4 cups water

2 medium red bell peppers, cut into 1-inch squares

1 cup chopped onion

2/3 cup uncooked brown rice

1/2 teaspoon ground turmeric

1/4 teaspoon crushed red pepper flakes

1/2 cup chopped fresh parsley

1 tablespoon olive oil (extra virgin preferred)

1/4 teaspoon salt

Exchanges / Choices
1 Starch, 1 Vegetable, 1/2 Fat

Calories	120	Sodium	75 mg
Calories from Fat	30	Potassium	210 mg
Total Fat	**3 g**	**Total Carbohydrate**	**21 g**
Saturated Fat	0.5 g	Dietary Fiber	2 g
Trans Fat	0 g	Sugars	3 g
Polyunsaturated Fat	0.5 g	**Protein**	**2 g**
Monounsaturated Fat	2 g	**Phosphorus**	**75 mg**
Cholesterol	**0 mg**		

1. In a medium saucepan, bring the water to a boil over high heat. Stir in the bell peppers, onion, rice, turmeric, and red pepper flakes. Return to a boil. Reduce the heat and simmer, covered, for 40 minutes, or until the rice is tender and the liquid is absorbed. Remove from the heat.

2. Stir in the parsley, oil, and salt.

ITALIAN SKILLET SPINACH

Serves 4 / Serving Size: 1/2 cup

All it takes is one minute from the time the spinach hits the skillet until the time it hits the serving bowl. Speed cooking brings you lightly seasoned spinach at its freshest. The heat of the red pepper flakes contrasts perfectly with the zing of lemon and earthiness of oregano.

2 tablespoons light tub margarine

1 teaspoon grated lemon zest

1 teaspoon dried oregano, crumbled

1/8 teaspoon crushed red pepper flakes

1/8 teaspoon salt

9 ounces spinach

3 tablespoons water

Exchanges / Choices			
1 Vegetable, 1/2 Fat			
Calories	40	Sodium	180 mg
Calories from Fat	30	Potassium	360 mg
Total Fat	3 g	Total Carbohydrate	3 g
Saturated Fat	0.5 g	Dietary Fiber	2 g
Trans Fat	0 g	Sugars	0 g
Polyunsaturated Fat	1 g	Protein	2 g
Monounsaturated Fat	1 g	Phosphorus	30 mg
Cholesterol	0 mg		

1. In a small bowl, stir together the margarine, lemon zest, oregano, red pepper flakes, and salt.

2. In a large nonstick skillet, cook the spinach and water over medium-high heat for 1 minute, or until tender, using two utensils to toss constantly. Remove from the heat.

3. Stir in the margarine mixture.

Cook's Tip: Fresh spinach cooks down rapidly. Toss or stir it constantly so it will cook evenly.

ACORN SQUASH WITH DRIED APRICOTS AND PLUMS

Serves 4 / Serving Size: 1/2 squash

Sweet, nutty acorn squash halves cradle a rich mixture of dried fruits and spices bound together with a juicy sauce, providing a beautiful and festive touch for a holiday table or a Sunday dinner. But they're so easy to prepare, they can make any night seem special.

Cooking spray

2 acorn squash (about 1 pound each), halved, seeds and strings discarded

1/2 cup dried apricots, chopped

1/4 cup orange-flavor dried plums, chopped

1/4 cup fresh orange juice

1 teaspoon ground cinnamon

1/4 teaspoon ground allspice or ground nutmeg

2 tablespoons light tub margarine

1. Preheat the oven to 350°F. Lightly spray a 13 × 9 × 2-inch baking dish with cooking spray.

2. Using a fork or the tip of a sharp knife, pierce the skin of the squash in several places. Put the squash with the cut side up in the baking dish.

3. In a small bowl, stir together the remaining ingredients except the margarine. Spoon into the squash cavities. Cover the pan with aluminum foil.

4. Bake for 1 hour 15 minutes, or until the squash is tender when the flesh is pierced with a fork. Remove from the oven.

5. Using a teaspoon, dot the margarine over the filling in each squash half. Let the margarine melt before serving the squash.

Cook's Tip: Kitchen scissors make it easy to snip the dried apricots and plums into small pieces. To prevent apricots and other dried fruits from sticking to the blades of the scissors, lightly spray the blades with cooking spray or run them under hot water and dry them just before you snip the fruit.

Exchanges / Choices
2 Starch, 1/2 Fruit

Calories	180	Sodium	50 mg
Calories from Fat	30	Potassium	1030 mg
Total Fat	**3.5 g**	**Total Carbohydrate**	**39 g**
Saturated Fat	0.5 g	Dietary Fiber	5 g
Trans Fat	0 g	Sugars	10 g
Polyunsaturated Fat	1 g	**Protein**	**3 g**
Monounsaturated Fat	1 g	**Phosphorus**	**95 mg**
Cholesterol	**0 mg**		

THYME-TINGED SQUASH

Serves 6 / Serving Size: 1/2 cup

A bit of sugar brings out the vegetables' natural sweetness and helps to caramelize them for an attractive presentation, turning simple summer squash and onion into something extraordinary. Try this with Citrus Chicken (page 73) or Mushroom-Smothered Cube Steak (page 93).

Cooking spray

1 pound yellow summer squash, sliced

1 large onion, chopped

1 teaspoon sugar

1/2 teaspoon dried thyme, crumbled

2 tablespoons light tub margarine

1/4 teaspoon salt

Exchanges / Choices
1 Vegetable

Calories	40	Sodium	100 mg
Calories from Fat	20	Potassium	230 mg
Total Fat	**2 g**	**Total Carbohydrate**	**5 g**
Saturated Fat	0.5 g	Dietary Fiber	1 g
Trans Fat	0 g	Sugars	3 g
Polyunsaturated Fat	0.5 g	**Protein**	**1 g**
Monounsaturated Fat	1 g	**Phosphorus**	**35 mg**
Cholesterol	**0 mg**		

1. Lightly spray a large skillet with cooking spray. Heat over medium-high heat. Remove from the heat. Put the squash, onion, sugar, and thyme in the skillet. Lightly spray the vegetables with cooking spray. Return to the heat and cook for 8 minutes, or until the squash is tender and beginning to richly brown, stirring frequently. Remove from the heat.

2. Stir in the margarine and salt.

LEMON-MINT SUGAR SNAPS

Serves 5 / Serving Size: 1/2 cup

The taste of delicate sugar snap peas teamed with fresh lemon and mint is definitely a harbinger of spring. Serve them with grilled or broiled lamb chops, or with a light fish dish, such as Tilapia with Dill and Paprika (page 56).

8 ounces sugar snap peas, trimmed

1/2 teaspoon grated lemon zest

2 tablespoons fresh lemon juice

1 tablespoon light tub margarine

1/8 teaspoon salt

1/4 cup chopped fresh mint or fresh cilantro

1. In a medium saucepan, steam the peas, covered, for 5 minutes, or until just tender-crisp. Drain well. Transfer to a medium bowl.

2. Meanwhile, in a small bowl, stir together the remaining ingredients except the mint.

3. Gently stir the lemon zest mixture and mint into the peas.

Exchanges / Choices
1 Vegetable

Calories	35	**Sodium**	55 mg
Calories from Fat	10	**Potassium**	100 mg
Total Fat	1 g	**Total Carbohydrate**	4 g
Saturated Fat	0.5 g	Dietary Fiber	1 g
Trans Fat	0 g	Sugars	2 g
Polyunsaturated Fat	0 g	**Protein**	1 g
Monounsaturated Fat	0.5 g	**Phosphorus**	25 mg
Cholesterol	0 mg		

BROWN-SUGAR-AND-SPICE SWEET POTATOES

Serves 4 / Serving Size: 1/2 sweet potato

A combination of dark brown sugar, warm spices, sweet vanilla, and creamy margarine melts over sweet potatoes for a delightfully aromatic side dish that will grace your autumn table. These are delicious alongside Roast Turkey with Orange-Spice Rub (page 83) or Onion-Smothered Pork Chops (page 109).

2 8-ounce sweet potatoes

1 1/2 tablespoons light tub margarine

1 tablespoon dark brown sugar

1/2 teaspoon grated orange zest

1/4 teaspoon ground cinnamon

1/4 teaspoon vanilla extract

1/8 teaspoon salt

Dash of ground allspice, ground nutmeg, or ground cloves

Exchanges / Choices
1 1/2 Starch

Calories	130	Sodium	95 mg
Calories from Fat	20	Potassium	400 mg
Total Fat	2 g	Total Carbohydrate	26 g
Saturated Fat	0.5 g	Dietary Fiber	4 g
Trans Fat	0 g	Sugars	8 g
Polyunsaturated Fat	0.5 g	Protein	2 g
Monounsaturated Fat	1 g	Phosphorus	55 mg
Cholesterol	0 mg		

1. Using a fork, pierce the skin of the sweet potatoes in several places. Place on a microwaveable plate or in a glass pie pan. Microwave on 100% power (high) for 8 minutes, or until the pulp is tender when pierced with a fork. Cut in half lengthwise. Fluff the pulp with a fork.

2. Meanwhile, in a small bowl, stir together the remaining ingredients.

3. Spoon the margarine mixture over the sweet potatoes.

TARRAGON TOMATOES

Serves 4 / Serving Size: 1 tomato

By using this mayo-mustard topping to heighten the flavor of tomatoes, you can enjoy them all year round. The small amount of horseradish adds just enough sharpness to contrast with the sweet-tart flavor of the tomatoes and the anise-like taste of tarragon.

2 tablespoons light mayonnaise

1 1/2 teaspoons Dijon mustard (lowest sodium available)

1 teaspoon bottled white horseradish, drained

1/2 teaspoon dried tarragon, crumbled

4 medium tomatoes, 1/4-inch slices cut from the stem ends and very thin slices cut from the bottoms

1/3 cup soft whole-wheat bread crumbs (lowest sodium available)

Olive oil cooking spray

Exchanges / Choices	
2 Vegetable	

Calories	50	**Sodium**	130 mg
Calories from Fat	20	**Potassium**	310 mg
Total Fat	**2 g**	**Total Carbohydrate**	**8 g**
Saturated Fat	0.5 g	Dietary Fiber	2 g
Trans Fat	0 g	Sugars	4 g
Polyunsaturated Fat	1 g	**Protein**	**2 g**
Monounsaturated Fat	0.5 g	**Phosphorus**	36 mg
Cholesterol	**<5 mg**		

1. Preheat the oven to 350°F.

2. In a small bowl, whisk together the mayonnaise, mustard, horseradish, and tarragon.

3. Place the tomatoes with the stem end up in a pie pan. Spread the mayonnaise mixture over each tomato. Top with the bread crumbs. Lightly spray the crumbs with cooking spray.

4. Bake for 30 minutes, or until the tomatoes are just tender when pierced with a fork. Remove from the oven. Let stand for 5 minutes before serving.

Cook's Tip: Cutting that very thin slice off the bottom of each tomato keeps the tomatoes from tilting and losing their tasty topping. Be careful not to cut too deep, or you'll allow too much juice to escape.

MEDITERRANEAN ZUCCHINI

Serves 4 / Serving Size: 1/2 zucchini

With its sunny seasonings of fresh lemon zest, basil, oregano, and red pepper flakes, this recipe pays homage to the humble zucchini and elevates it to a whole new level of deliciousness. Bake it alongside Salmon Baked with Cucumbers and Dill (page 52) or Baked Parmesan Chicken (page 68).

2 medium zucchini (5–6 ounces each), trimmed and halved lengthwise

2 teaspoons olive oil

1/2 teaspoon grated lemon zest

1/2 teaspoon dried basil, crumbled

1/2 teaspoon dried oregano, crumbled

1/8 teaspoon crushed red pepper flakes

1/8 teaspoon salt

1 tablespoon plus 1 teaspoon shredded or grated Parmesan cheese

Exchanges / Choices
1 Vegetable, 1/2 Fat

Calories	40	**Sodium**	80 mg
Calories from Fat	30	**Potassium**	230 mg
Total Fat	3 g	**Total Carbohydrate**	3 g
Saturated Fat	0.5 g	Dietary Fiber	1 g
Trans Fat	0 g	Sugars	2 g
Polyunsaturated Fat	0.5 g	**Protein**	2 g
Monounsaturated Fat	2 g	**Phosphorus**	45 mg
Cholesterol	<5 mg		

1. Preheat the oven to 400°F.

2. Place the zucchini with the cut side up on a baking sheet. Drizzle the oil over each half.

3. In a small bowl, stir together the remaining ingredients except the Parmesan. Sprinkle over the zucchini.

4. Bake for 20 minutes, or until the zucchini is just tender. Remove from the oven.

5. Sprinkle with the Parmesan. Let stand for 5 minutes before serving.

VEGGIE STIR-FRY, MEXICAN STYLE

Serves 5 / Serving Size: 1/2 cup

Great with broiled or skillet-grilled chicken or pork, this side dish medley of carrots, onion, and corn gets some spicy Mexican flair from strips of poblano, chili powder, and cumin.

Cooking spray

1 medium poblano pepper or 1 medium green bell pepper, seeds and ribs discarded, cut into thin strips

1/2 cup matchstick-size carrot strips

1/2 medium onion, thinly sliced

1 1/2 cups frozen whole-kernel corn, thawed, drained, and patted dry with paper towels

1 1/2 tablespoons light tub margarine

1/2 teaspoon chili powder

1/2 teaspoon ground cumin

1/4 teaspoon dried oregano, crumbled

1/8 teaspoon salt

1/8 teaspoon crushed red pepper flakes

Exchanges / Choices

1/2 Starch, 1 Vegetable

Calories	90	**Sodium**	60 mg
Calories from Fat	25	**Potassium**	250 mg
Total Fat	2.5 g	**Total Carbohydrate**	16 g
Saturated Fat	0.5 g	Dietary Fiber	2 g
Trans Fat	0 g	Sugars	4 g
Polyunsaturated Fat	1 g	**Protein**	2 g
Monounsaturated Fat	1 g	**Phosphorus**	50 mg
Cholesterol	0 mg		

1. Lightly spray a large skillet with cooking spray. Heat over medium-high heat. Cook the poblano, carrot, and onion for 7–8 minutes, or until beginning to brown on the edges, stirring frequently.

2. Stir in the corn. Cook for 1 minute, stirring frequently. Remove from the heat.

3. Stir in the remaining ingredients.

NUTMEG-SPICED VEGETABLE MEDLEY

Serves 4 / Serving Size: 2/3 cup

Nutmeg and cumin blend to provide a mildly spiced seasoning for a trio of steamed vegetables whose bright colors will perk up any plate while letting the entrée star.

1 cup sliced carrots

1 cup cauliflower florets

1 cup broccoli florets

2 tablespoons light tub margarine

1 teaspoon sugar

1/4 teaspoon ground cumin

1/8 teaspoon salt

1/8 teaspoon ground nutmeg

Dash of cayenne

Exchanges / Choices
1 Vegetable, 1/2 Fat

Calories	50	Sodium	190 mg
Calories from Fat	30	Potassium	190 mg
Total Fat	**3 g**	**Total Carbohydrate**	**5 g**
Saturated Fat	0.5 g	Dietary Fiber	1 g
Trans Fat	0 g	Sugars	3 g
Polyunsaturated Fat	1 g	**Protein**	**1 g**
Monounsaturated Fat	1 g	**Phosphorus**	**30 mg**
Cholesterol	**0 mg**		

1. In a medium saucepan, steam the carrots, cauliflower, and broccoli, covered, for 5 minutes, or until just tender-crisp. Drain well. Transfer to a medium bowl.

2. Meanwhile, in a small bowl, stir together the remaining ingredients.

3. Stir the margarine mixture into the carrot mixture.

| *Breads and Breakfast* |

ROSEMARY QUICK BREAD

Serves 16 / Serving Size: 1 slice

Even the novice cook can prepare this savory bread with confidence. It goes together quickly, requires no rising time, and will perfume your house with the fragrance of rosemary and garlic as it bakes.

Cooking spray

2 cups all-purpose flour

1 cup whole-wheat flour

1 teaspoon dried rosemary, crushed

1 teaspoon baking soda

1/2 teaspoon baking powder

1/2 teaspoon garlic powder

1/2 teaspoon salt

1 1/3 cups low-fat buttermilk

3 tablespoons honey

2 tablespoons olive oil

1. Preheat the oven to 350°F. Lightly spray a baking sheet with cooking spray.

2. In a large bowl, stir together both flours, the rosemary, baking soda, baking powder, garlic powder, and salt.

3. Add the buttermilk, honey, and oil, stirring only until the dough is moistened.

4. Shape the dough into a ball. Put the dough on a flat surface and knead gently for about 5 seconds. Put the dough on the baking sheet. Shape the dough into an oval loaf, about 8 × 6 inches. Slightly flatten the top. Using a sharp knife, cut 4 diagonal slices about 1/4 inch deep across the top of the bread. These will prevent the loaf from cracking during baking.

5. Bake for 40–45 minutes, or until the loaf is golden brown, sounds hollow when tapped, and registers 190°F on an instant-read thermometer. Remove from the baking sheet and transfer to a cooling rack. Let cool for 10–15 minutes before slicing.

Exchanges / Choices
1 1/2 Starch

Calories	120	Sodium	170 mg
Calories from Fat	25	Potassium	80 mg
Total Fat	2.5 g	Total Carbohydrate	22 g
Saturated Fat	0 g	Dietary Fiber	1 g
Trans Fat	0 g	Sugars	4 g
Polyunsaturated Fat	0.5 g	Protein	3 g
Monounsaturated Fat	1.5 g	Phosphorus	65 mg
Cholesterol	<5 mg		

LEMON-LIME POPPY SEED MUFFINS

Serves 12 / Serving Size: 1 muffin

Moist and satisfying with the delicate crunch of poppy seeds and the brightness of citrus, these muffins are a surefire way to start your morning on the right track.

Cooking spray

2 cups all-purpose flour

1/2 cup firmly packed light brown sugar

1 tablespoon poppy seeds

2 teaspoons baking powder

1/2 teaspoon baking soda

1/4 teaspoon salt

1 cup fat-free milk

1 large egg

2 tablespoons honey

1 tablespoon canola or corn oil

2 teaspoons grated lemon zest

1 tablespoon fresh lemon juice

2 teaspoons grated lime zest

1. Preheat the oven to 375°F. Lightly spray a standard 12-cup muffin pan with cooking spray.

2. In a large bowl, stir together the flour, brown sugar, poppy seeds, baking powder, baking soda, and salt. Make a well in the center of the mixture.

3. In a small bowl, whisk together the remaining ingredients. Pour into the well, stirring until the batter is just moistened but no flour is visible. Don't overmix; the batter will be slightly lumpy. Put about 1/4 cup batter in each muffin cup.

4. Bake for 15–17 minutes, or until a wooden toothpick inserted in the center of a muffin comes out clean. Transfer the pan to a cooling rack and let cool for 10 minutes before removing the muffins from the pan.

Exchanges / Choices

1 1/2 Carbohydrate

Calories	140	**Sodium**	180 mg
Calories from Fat	20	**Potassium**	80 mg
Total Fat	2 g	**Total Carbohydrate**	26 g
Saturated Fat	0.5 g	Dietary Fiber	1 g
Trans Fat	0 g	Sugars	10 g
Polyunsaturated Fat	0.5 g	**Protein**	4 g
Monounsaturated Fat	1 g	**Phosphorus**	75 mg
Cholesterol	15 mg		

APRICOT AND APPLE GRANOLA

Serves 16 / Serving Size: 1/2 cup

Making your own homemade granola is easy. Make it a family project and let everyone help measure, mix, and bake. Then pack the cooled mixture into small airtight plastic bags for a quick breakfast or snack on the go.

Cooking spray

4 cups uncooked quick-cooking oatmeal

1/2 cup toasted wheat germ

1/2 cup firmly packed light brown sugar

1/4 cup sliced almonds

1 teaspoon ground cinnamon

1/2 cup water

1/2 cup 100% apricot nectar or juice

2 tablespoons honey

1 tablespoon canola or corn oil

2 cups bran cereal (buds or flakes)

1/2 cup chopped dried apricots

1/2 cup chopped dried apples

1. Preheat the oven to 300°F. Lightly spray a rimmed baking sheet with cooking spray.

2. In a large bowl, stir together the oatmeal, wheat germ, brown sugar, almonds, and cinnamon.

3. In a small bowl, whisk together the water, apricot nectar, honey, and oil. Pour into the oatmeal mixture. Stir until all the mixture is moistened. Spread on the baking sheet.

4. Bake for 1 hour, or until the mixture is toasted and lightly golden brown, stirring every 20 minutes. Transfer the baking sheet to a cooling rack. Let the mixture cool for 30 minutes. Transfer to a large bowl. Stir in the bran cereal, apricots, and apples.

Cook's Tip: While the granola is still warm, try some with fat-free milk poured on top. Then store what's left in an airtight container or airtight plastic bags at room temperature for up to two weeks.

Exchanges / Choices
2 Carbohydrate, 1/2 Fat

Calories	170	Sodium	50 mg
Calories from Fat	30	Potassium	220 mg
Total Fat	**3.5 g**	**Total Carbohydrate**	**32 g**
Saturated Fat	0.5 g	Dietary Fiber	4 g
Trans Fat	0 g	Sugars	12 g
Polyunsaturated Fat	0 g	**Protein**	**5 g**
Monounsaturated Fat	0 g	**Phosphorus**	**160 mg**
Cholesterol	**0 mg**		

CHERRY OATMEAL

Serves 4 / Serving Size: 1 cup

Warm, comforting, and healthy, too—a bowl of oatmeal is all those things. You won't even think about adding sugar and milk once you've tasted how the cherries and yogurt enrich this fruity breakfast dish that's ready in a snap.

3 1/2 cups water

1/2 cup sweetened dried cherries

2 cups uncooked quick-cooking oatmeal

6 ounces fat-free vanilla yogurt

1. In a medium saucepan, bring the water and cherries to a boil, covered, over medium-high heat. Reduce the heat to low and cook, uncovered, for 5 minutes, stirring occasionally.

2. Stir in the oatmeal. Cook for 1–2 minutes, or until the oatmeal is thickened, stirring occasionally. Spoon into bowls. Dollop each serving with the yogurt. Using the tip of a flat knife, such as a butter knife, swirl the yogurt through the oatmeal.

Exchanges / Choices

1 Fruit, 2 Starch

Calories	220	**Sodium**	35 mg
Calories from Fat	25	**Potassium**	280 mg
Total Fat	**2.5 g**	**Total Carbohydrate**	**46 g**
Saturated Fat	0.5 g	Dietary Fiber	5 g
Trans Fat	0 g	Sugars	15 g
Polyunsaturated Fat	1 g	**Protein**	**7 g**
Monounsaturated Fat	1 g	**Phosphorus**	**210 mg**
Cholesterol	**<5 mg**		

FARMERS' MARKET OMELETS

Serves 4 / Serving Size: 1/2 omelet

Brighten up your breakfast with these flavorful omelets, full of fresh vegetables, fragrant basil, and pungent feta cheese. Add some whole-grain toast and fresh fruit for a light, nutritious meal any time of day. *(See photo insert.)*

1 tablespoon plus 1 teaspoon canola or corn oil, divided use

1 cup grape tomatoes, halved

1 cup baby spinach

6 large egg whites

2 large eggs

1/4 cup fat-free milk

4 medium green onions, chopped

1/4 cup chopped fresh basil

2 ounces fat-free feta cheese, crumbled

1. In a medium nonstick skillet, heat 2 teaspoons oil over medium heat, swirling to coat the bottom. Cook the tomatoes and spinach for 2–3 minutes, or until the tomatoes are slightly softened, stirring constantly. Transfer the mixture to a plate. Cover to keep warm. Set aside. Wipe the skillet with paper towels.

2. In a small bowl, using a fork, lightly beat together the egg whites, eggs, and milk. Stir in the green onions.

3. In the same skillet, still over medium heat, heat 1 teaspoon oil, swirling to coat the bottom. Pour half the egg white mixture into the skillet, swirling to coat the bottom. Cook for 30 seconds, or until beginning to set. Using a spatula, carefully lift the cooked edge of the omelet and tilt the skillet so the uncooked portion flows under the edge. Cook until no runniness remains, repeating the lift-and-tilt procedure once or twice at other places along the edge if needed.

4. With the skillet still on the burner, spread half the tomato mixture over half the omelet. Sprinkle, in order, with half the basil and half the feta. Remove from the heat. Using a spatula, carefully fold the half with no filling over the other half. Cut the omelet in half crosswise. Gently slide onto plates. Cover to keep warm.

5. Using the remaining ingredients, including the final 1 teaspoon oil, make and fill a second omelet.

Cook's Tip: Although these omelets are top-notch with basil, feel free to use a different fresh herb or combine several for even more subtle layers of fresh flavor.

Exchanges / Choices			
1 Vegetable, 2 Lean Meat			

Calories	130	Sodium	290 mg
Calories from Fat	50	Potassium	350 mg
Total Fat	**6 g**	**Total Carbohydrate**	**6 g**
Saturated Fat	1 g	Dietary Fiber	1 g
Trans Fat	0 g	Sugars	4 g
Polyunsaturated Fat	1.5 g	**Protein**	**12 g**
Monounsaturated Fat	3 g	**Phosphorus**	**140 mg**
Cholesterol	**100 mg**		

SOUTHWESTERN BREAKFAST TORTILLA WRAPS

Serves 6 / Serving Size: 1 wrap

Make a batch of the filling ahead of time so you can microwave one portion at a time for a warm, filling breakfast before you head out the door. Just zap, wrap, and go.

4 ounces low-fat turkey breakfast sausage links, casings discarded

Cooking spray

2 cups frozen whole-kernel corn

4 large egg whites

2 large eggs

1/4 teaspoon chili powder

6 (6-inch) fat-free whole-grain tortillas

1/4 cup salsa (lowest sodium available)

1/4 cup shredded fat-free cheddar cheese

1. Heat a medium nonstick skillet over medium-high heat. Cook the sausage for 6–8 minutes, or until cooked through, stirring to break up the turkey. Transfer the sausage to a plate. Set aside. Wipe the skillet with paper towels.

2. Meanwhile, lightly spray the same skillet with cooking spray. Reduce the heat to medium. Cook the corn for 4–5 minutes, or until heated through, stirring occasionally.

3. In a small bowl, using a fork, lightly beat together the egg whites, eggs, and chili powder. Stir the egg white mixture into the corn. Cook for 3–4 minutes, or until the egg white mixture is cooked through, stirring occasionally. Stir in the sausage.

4. Warm the tortillas using the package directions.

5. Spoon 1/2 cup egg white mixture down the center of each tortilla. Top with the salsa. Sprinkle with the cheddar. Fold the bottom, then the sides, then the top of each tortilla toward the center. Place with the seam side down on a plate.

Cook's Tip: Store the extra filling, covered, in the refrigerator for up to three days. Microwave one serving on 100% power (high) for 30 seconds to 1 minute. Assemble the wrap as directed.

Exchanges / Choices
1 1/2 Starch, 1 Lean Meat

Calories	180	**Sodium**	330 mg
Calories from Fat	35	**Potassium**	270 mg
Total Fat	4 g	**Total Carbohydrate**	26 g
Saturated Fat	1 g	Dietary Fiber	2 g
Trans Fat	0 g	Sugars	2 g
Polyunsaturated Fat	1 g	**Protein**	11 g
Monounsaturated Fat	1.5 g	**Phosphorus**	125 mg
Cholesterol	70 mg		

APPLE PIE BREAKFAST PARFAITS

Serves 6 / Serving Size: 1 parfait

Apple pie for breakfast? When cinnamon-scented apple slices are layered with vanilla yogurt, then topped with golden raisins and dry-roasted walnuts, this crustless version fits the bill.

1 (20-ounce) can unsweetened sliced apples, drained

1 tablespoon honey

1 teaspoon grated lemon zest

1 teaspoon fresh lemon juice

1/2 teaspoon ground cinnamon

4 cups fat-free vanilla yogurt

1/4 cup golden raisins

3 tablespoons chopped walnuts, dry-roasted

Exchanges / Choices			
1 Fruit, 1 Fat-Free Milk			

Calories	170	**Sodium**	90 mg
Calories from Fat	30	**Potassium**	420 mg
Total Fat	**3 g**	**Total Carbohydrate**	**32 g**
Saturated Fat	0 g	Dietary Fiber	2 g
Trans Fat	0 g	Sugars	27 g
Polyunsaturated Fat	1.5 g	**Protein**	**7 g**
Monounsaturated Fat	1 g	**Phosphorus**	200 mg
Cholesterol	**<5 mg**		

1. In a small bowl, stir together the apples, honey, lemon zest, lemon juice, and cinnamon.

2. In a parfait glass or other tall clear glass, layer the ingredients as follows: 2 1/2 table-spoons apple mixture, then 1/3 cup yogurt. Repeat the layers. Sprinkle each parfait with the raisins and walnuts.

APPLE CRUMBLE COFFEE CAKE

Serves 16 / Serving Size: one 2-inch square

Coffee cake with a crisp crumbled topping and a surprise of moist, tender apples on the bottom—what a lovely way to begin your day!

Cooking spray

2 medium Granny Smith apples, peeled and thinly sliced

2 tablespoons 100% apple juice

1 tablespoon honey

1 teaspoon ground cinnamon

1 1/2 cups all-purpose flour

1/3 cup sugar

2 1/2 teaspoons baking powder

1/2 cup fat-free milk

1/4 cup unsweetened applesauce

1/4 cup egg substitute or 1 large egg

1 tablespoon canola or corn oil

1/2 cup uncooked quick-cooking oatmeal

3 tablespoons light brown sugar

3 tablespoons chopped pecans

2 tablespoons light tub margarine, softened

1 teaspoon ground cinnamon

1. Preheat the oven to 375°F. Lightly spray an 8-inch square baking dish with cooking spray. Set aside.

2. In a medium nonstick skillet, cook the apples and apple juice over medium heat for 4–5 minutes, or until the apples are tender-crisp, stirring occasionally.

3. Stir in the honey and cinnamon. Cook for 1–2 minutes, or until the cinnamon is distributed throughout the apples and the mixture is heated through, stirring occasionally.

4. Put the baking dish on a cooling rack. Pour the apple mixture into the pan. Let cool for 5 minutes.

5. In a medium bowl, stir together the flour, sugar, and baking powder. Make a well in the center. Add the milk, applesauce, egg substitute, and oil to the well, stirring until the batter is just moistened but no flour is visible. Don't overmix; the batter will be slightly lumpy. Pour the batter over the apple mixture.

6. In a small bowl, using a fork, stir together the remaining ingredients. Sprinkle over the batter.

7. Bake for 25–30 minutes, or until a wooden toothpick inserted in the center comes out clean. Transfer the dish to a cooling rack. Let cool for 15 minutes before cutting into squares.

Exchanges / Choices	
1 1/2 Carbohydrate	

Calories	120	**Sodium**	100 mg
Calories from Fat	30	**Potassium**	90 mg
Total Fat	**3 g**	**Total Carbohydrate**	**22 g**
Saturated Fat	0 g	Dietary Fiber	1 g
Trans Fat	0 g	Sugars	10 g
Polyunsaturated Fat	1 g	**Protein**	**2 g**
Monounsaturated Fat	1.5 g	**Phosphorus**	**60 mg**
Cholesterol	**<5 mg**		

FRENCH TOAST CASSEROLE WITH HONEY-GLAZED FRUIT

Serves 6 / Serving Size: 2/3 cup

Make weekend mornings special with this lightly sweetened French toast casserole. It may taste decadent, but each serving provides protein from egg substitute and fat-free milk, fiber from whole-wheat bread, and even fruit. *(See photo insert.)*

Cooking spray

6 slices whole-wheat bread (lowest sodium available), halved lengthwise

1 1/2 cups fat-free milk

1 1/2 cups egg substitute

2 tablespoons light brown sugar

1 teaspoon ground cinnamon

1/4 teaspoon ground nutmeg

1 (15-ounce) can light fruit cocktail, drained

2 tablespoons honey

1 tablespoon light tub margarine

1. Preheat the oven to 350°F. Lightly spray an 8-inch square baking dish with cooking spray.

2. Place the bread halves with the cut sides (the crustless sides) touching the bottom of the pan and the crust sides resting on the slice beneath them. The slices should overlap slightly. Set aside.

3. In a medium bowl, whisk together the milk, egg substitute, brown sugar, cinnamon, and nutmeg. Pour over the bread. Using a spoon, press down the bread to soak up the milk mixture. Spread the fruit cocktail over the bread. Drizzle with the honey. Using a teaspoon, dot with the margarine.

4. Bake for 55 minutes–1 hour, or until the center of the casserole is set (doesn't jiggle when the casserole is gently shaken). Let cool for at least 10 minutes before cutting.

Cook's Tip: If you prepare this casserole ahead of time, cover it with plastic wrap and refrigerate for up to 10 hours. Uncover it, put the cold casserole in a cold oven, set the temperature to 350°F, and bake for 1 hour 5 minutes–1 hour 10 minutes, or until the center is set (doesn't jiggle when the casserole is gently shaken). Let cool for at least 10 minutes before cutting.

Exchanges / Choices
2 Carbohydrate, 1 Lean Meat

Calories	180	**Sodium**	150 mg
Calories from Fat	30	**Potassium**	410 mg
Total Fat	3 g	**Total Carbohydrate**	27 g
Saturated Fat	0.5 g	Dietary Fiber	3 g
Trans Fat	0 g	Sugars	18 g
Polyunsaturated Fat	1 g	**Protein**	12 g
Monounsaturated Fat	1 g	**Phosphorus**	190 mg
Cholesterol	<5 mg		

| *Desserts* |

COCOA APPLESAUCE CAKE

Serves 24 / Serving Size: one 1 3/4-inch square

This cake's powerfully rich taste comes from unsweetened cocoa powder. Oatmeal adds a boost of fiber, while low-fat buttermilk and applesauce make it plenty moist!

Cooking spray

1 1/4 cups whole-wheat pastry flour or all-purpose flour

1/3 cup sugar

1/3 cup unsweetened Dutch process cocoa powder

1/4 cup uncooked regular or quick-cooking oatmeal

1 1/2 teaspoons baking powder

1 teaspoon baking soda

1 cup low-fat buttermilk

2/3 cup unsweetened applesauce

1/2 cup egg substitute or 2 large eggs

3 tablespoons canola or corn oil

1 teaspoon vanilla extract

1. Preheat the oven to 350°F. Lightly spray an 11 × 7 × 2-inch glass baking dish with cooking spray.

2. In a medium bowl, stir together the flour, sugar, cocoa, oatmeal, baking powder, and baking soda.

3. In a large bowl, whisk together the remaining ingredients. Stir the flour mixture into the buttermilk mixture until the batter is just moistened but no flour is visible. Spread the batter in the baking dish, gently smoothing the top.

4. Bake for 40–45 minutes, or until the cake springs back when gently touched in the center and a wooden toothpick inserted in the center comes out clean. Transfer the dish to a cooling rack. Let cool completely before cutting the cake into squares.

Cook's Tip on Cocoa Powder: Dutch process cocoa powder, sometimes referred to as dark cocoa powder, has been treated with alkaline to reduce the cocoa's natural acidity. It has a smoother, less bitter taste and a deeper, less reddish hue.

Exchanges / Choices
1 Carbohydrate

Calories	70	**Sodium**	105 mg
Calories from Fat	25	**Potassium**	80 mg
Total Fat	**2.5 g**	**Total Carbohydrate**	**10 g**
Saturated Fat	0.5 g	Dietary Fiber	1 g
Trans Fat	0 g	Sugars	4 g
Polyunsaturated Fat	0.5 g	**Protein**	**2 g**
Monounsaturated Fat	1.5 g	**Phosphorus**	40 mg
Cholesterol	**<5 mg**		

MINI CHOCOLATE-RASPBERRY SHORTCAKES

Serves 6 / Serving Size: 1 shortcake

Shortcake, one of America's favorite desserts, is given a twist when we top a dark chocolate version with fresh raspberries in yogurt and whipped topping.

3/4 cup all-purpose flour

1/4 cup unsweetened cocoa powder (Dutch process preferred)

1/4 cup sugar

1 1/2 teaspoons baking powder

3/4 cup fat-free, sugar-free vanilla yogurt, divided use

1/4 cup fat-free milk

1 tablespoon canola or corn oil

1 1/2 cups raspberries

1/4 cup plus 2 tablespoons refrigerated fat-free aerosol whipped topping

1. Preheat the oven to 450°F. Line a baking sheet with parchment paper.

2. In a small bowl, stir together the flour, cocoa, sugar, and baking powder. In a separate small bowl, whisk together 1/4 cup yogurt, the milk, and oil until smooth. Stir the yogurt mixture into the flour mixture until the batter is just moistened but no flour is visible. Don't overmix; the batter should be slightly lumpy. Spoon six 1/4-cup mounds of batter onto the baking sheet.

3. Bake for 8–10 minutes, or until a wooden toothpick inserted in the center of a mound comes out clean or with only a few moist crumbs. Transfer the baking sheet to a cooling rack and let cool for 20–30 minutes, or until room temperature or slightly warm.

4. Just before the shortcakes are cool, put the raspberries in a medium bowl. Gently stir in the remaining 1/2 cup yogurt.

5. Halve the shortcakes crosswise. Top each bottom half with the raspberry mixture. Put the top halves on. Dollop with the whipped topping.

Exchanges / Choices

2 Carbohydrate

Calories	140	**Sodium**	140 mg
Calories from Fat	15	**Potassium**	220 mg
Total Fat	**1.5 g**	**Total Carbohydrate**	**29 g**
Saturated Fat	1 g	Dietary Fiber	4 g
Trans Fat	0 g	Sugars	13 g
Polyunsaturated Fat	0 g	**Protein**	**4 g**
Monounsaturated Fat	0.5 g	**Phosphorus**	120 mg
Cholesterol	**<5 mg**		

PEACHES AND BERRIES CRISP

Serves 8 / Serving Size: 1/2 cup

A bounty of fruit makes this crisp irresistible. Only small amounts of honey and brown sugar are added so the natural sweetness of the fruit can shine brightly.

Cooking spray

2 cups fresh or frozen unsweetened sliced peaches, thawed if frozen

1 cup fresh or frozen unsweetened raspberries, thawed if frozen

1 cup fresh or frozen unsweetened blueberries, thawed if frozen

2 tablespoons honey (1 tablespoon if using frozen peaches)

1 teaspoon grated lemon zest

1 teaspoon fresh lemon juice

1/4 teaspoon ground nutmeg

1 cup uncooked quick-cooking oatmeal

1/4 cup whole-wheat flour or all-purpose flour

1/4 cup chopped walnuts, dry-roasted

3 tablespoons light brown sugar

2 tablespoons light tub margarine, at room temperature

1 teaspoon ground cinnamon

1. Preheat the oven to 350°F. Lightly spray an 8-inch square baking dish with cooking spray.

2. Place the peaches, raspberries, blueberries, honey, lemon zest, lemon juice, and nutmeg in the baking dish, stirring gently 4 or 5 times, being careful not to break up the raspberries.

3. In a medium bowl, stir together the remaining ingredients until the margarine is distributed throughout. Sprinkle over the peach mixture.

4. Bake for 25–30 minutes, or until the top of the crisp is golden brown.

Exchanges / Choices
1 Carbohydrate, 1 Fruit, 1 Fat

Calories	170	Sodium	25 mg
Calories from Fat	45	Potassium	180 mg
Total Fat	5 g	Total Carbohydrate	30 g
Saturated Fat	1 g	Dietary Fiber	4 g
Trans Fat	0 g	Sugars	17 g
Polyunsaturated Fat	2.5 g	Protein	3 g
Monounsaturated Fat	1 g	Phosphorus	85 mg
Cholesterol	0 mg		

COCOA-ALMOND KISSES WITH ORANGE ZEST

Serves 20 / Serving Size: 2 cookies

These little gems are crunchy on the outside and chewy on the inside. The delectable flavors of cocoa and almonds—plus a light tang from snippets of orange zest—permeate every bite.

Cooking spray (optional)

1/2 cup sugar

3 tablespoons unsweetened cocoa powder (Dutch process preferred)

3 large egg whites, at room temperature

1/4 teaspoon cream of tartar

1 teaspoon grated orange zest

1/2 teaspoon almond extract

1/2 cup slivered almonds, dry-roasted and finely chopped

1. Preheat the oven to 275°F. Lightly spray a large baking sheet with cooking spray, or line it with parchment paper or aluminum foil.

2. In a small bowl, stir together the sugar and cocoa.

3. In a large mixing bowl, using an electric mixer on medium-high speed, beat the egg whites and cream of tartar until foamy. Gradually add the sugar mixture to the egg white mixture, continuing to beat until the batter is shiny and forms stiff peaks.

4. Using a plastic or rubber spatula, gently fold in the orange zest, almond extract, and almonds.

5. Drop the batter by rounded teaspoons onto the baking sheet, leaving a 1-inch space between the meringues.

6. Bake for 40 minutes, or until the meringues are firm. Turn off the oven. Let the meringues dry, with the oven door closed, for 30 minutes. Transfer the baking sheet to a cooling rack and let cool completely. Store the meringues in an airtight container for up to one week.

Cook's Tip: Room temperature egg whites will produce more volume when whipped than will egg whites straight from the refrigerator. Either take the eggs out ahead of time or briefly place them in a bowl of hot water until they come to room temperature. Adding a bit of cream of tartar to the whites also helps to increase the volume. Even a single drop of egg yolk will prevent egg whites from forming peaks when beaten, so separate eggs very carefully.

Exchanges / Choices
1/2 Carbohydrate

Calories	40	Sodium	10 mg
Calories from Fat	15	Potassium	45 mg
Total Fat	**1.5 g**	**Total Carbohydrate**	**6 g**
Saturated Fat	0 g	Dietary Fiber	1 g
Trans Fat	0 g	Sugars	5 g
Polyunsaturated Fat	0.5 g	**Protein**	**1 g**
Monounsaturated Fat	1 g	**Phosphorus**	**20 mg**
Cholesterol	**0 mg**		

APPLESAUCE-ALMOND SQUARES

Serves 24 / Serving Size: one 1 3/4-inch square

Ground almonds in the dry ingredients, almond extract in the batter, and slivered almonds on the top give these tender bars a wonderfully nutty taste. Applesauce provides flavor, moistness, and natural sweetness.

Cooking spray

1 cup unsweetened applesauce

1/2 cup fat-free milk

1/3 cup fat-free plain yogurt

2 large egg whites

3 tablespoons canola or corn oil

1/2 teaspoon almond extract

1 cup whole-wheat pastry flour or all-purpose flour

1/4 cup plus 2 tablespoons firmly packed dark brown sugar

1/4 cup uncooked regular or quick-cooking oatmeal

1/4 cup ground or finely chopped almonds

1 1/2 teaspoons baking powder

1/2 teaspoon ground cinnamon

1/4 teaspoon ground cardamom

1/8 teaspoon salt

3 tablespoons slivered almonds

1. Preheat the oven to 350°F. Lightly spray an 11 x 7 x 2-inch baking dish with cooking spray.

2. In a large bowl, whisk together the applesauce, milk, yogurt, egg whites, oil, and almond extract.

3. In a medium bowl, stir together the remaining ingredients except the slivered almonds. Stir the flour mixture into the applesauce mixture until the batter is just moistened but no flour is visible. Spread the batter in the baking dish, gently smoothing the top. Sprinkle with the slivered almonds.

4. Bake for 35–38 minutes, or until a wooden toothpick inserted in the center comes out clean. Transfer the dish to a cooling rack and let cool completely before cutting into squares.

Cook's Tip: For baking, whole-wheat pastry flour is preferable to regular whole-wheat flour because the pastry flour is finer in texture and produces a more tender finished product. You can usually find whole-wheat pastry flour with the other flour and baking ingredients in the baking aisle of your supermarket.

Exchanges / Choices
1 Carbohydrate

Calories	70	**Sodium**	50 mg
Calories from Fat	30	**Potassium**	60 mg
Total Fat	**3 g**	**Total Carbohydrate**	**10 g**
Saturated Fat	0 g	Dietary Fiber	1 g
Trans Fat	0 g	Sugars	5 g
Polyunsaturated Fat	1 g	**Protein**	**2 g**
Monounsaturated Fat	1.5 g	**Phosphorus**	**35 mg**
Cholesterol	**<5 mg**		

LEMON-RASPBERRY SQUARES

Serves 24 / Serving Size: one 1 3/4-inch square

These citrusy bars are loaded with the sweet-tart taste of fresh lemon and raspberries. Cornmeal adds a unique texture and a vibrant color to match the bright flavor.

Cooking spray

Zest from 1 medium lemon, 1 teaspoon zest transferred to a medium bowl and the remaining zest reserved

1 cup whole-wheat pastry flour or all-purpose flour

1/3 cup regular or quick-cooking oatmeal

1/3 cup yellow cornmeal

1/4 cup plus 2 tablespoons sugar

1 1/2 teaspoons baking powder

1/2 teaspoon baking soda

1/2 teaspoon ground cardamom

1/4 teaspoon ground cinnamon

1 cup low-fat buttermilk

2/3 cup unsweetened applesauce

1/2 cup egg substitute or 2 large eggs

3 tablespoons canola or corn oil

2 tablespoons fresh lemon juice

1 1/2 cups raspberries

1–2 tablespoons sifted confectioners' sugar

1. Preheat the oven to 350°F. Lightly spray an 11 x 7 x 2-inch glass baking dish with cooking spray.

2. In the medium bowl with the lemon zest, stir together the flour, oatmeal, cornmeal, sugar, baking powder, baking soda, cardamom, and cinnamon.

3. In a large bowl, whisk together the buttermilk, applesauce, egg substitute, oil, and lemon juice.

4. Stir the flour mixture into the buttermilk mixture until the batter is just moistened but no flour is visible. Gently fold in the raspberries. Spread the batter in the baking dish, gently smoothing the top.

5. Bake for 50–55 minutes, or until the top is springy to the touch and a wooden toothpick inserted in the center comes out clean. Transfer the dish to a cooling rack and let cool completely. Before cutting into squares, sprinkle with the confectioners' sugar and reserved lemon zest.

Cook's Tip: Cornmeal is used in place of some of the all-purpose flour in many Italian baked desserts. The cornmeal creates a more complex texture and adds dimension to the taste of the finished product.

Exchanges / Choices
1 Carbohydrate

Calories	80	**Sodium**	50 mg
Calories from Fat	25	**Potassium**	65 mg
Total Fat	2.5 g	**Total Carbohydrate**	12 g
Saturated Fat	0 g	Dietary Fiber	1 g
Trans Fat	0 g	Sugars	5 g
Polyunsaturated Fat	0.5 g	**Protein**	2 g
Monounsaturated Fat	1 g	**Phosphorus**	40 mg
Cholesterol	<5 mg		

ORANGE AND APPLE BARS

Serves 24 / Serving Size: one 1 3/4-inch square

These bars, with their thin layer of tasty apple butter, are a delightful snack or dessert. Make two batches at the same time, doubling the ingredients and using the oven just once, then freeze a batch for later.

Cooking spray

1 cup regular or quick-cooking oatmeal

1 cup whole-wheat pastry flour or all-purpose flour

1/4 cup sugar

1/2 teaspoon ground cardamom

1/4 teaspoon ground nutmeg

1/4 teaspoon baking soda

2 large egg whites

3 tablespoons canola or corn oil

2 teaspoons grated orange zest

2 tablespoons fresh orange juice

1 1/2 cups fruit butter, such as apple or pumpkin

1. Preheat the oven to 350°F. Lightly spray an 8-inch square baking dish with cooking spray.

2. In a medium bowl, stir together the oatmeal, flour, sugar, cardamom, nutmeg, and baking soda.

3. In a small bowl, using a fork, lightly beat the egg whites. Stir in the oil and orange juice.

4. Add the egg white mixture to the oatmeal mixture, stirring until the combined mixture holds together. Press three-fourths of the mixture into the baking dish.

5. In a medium bowl, whisk together the fruit butter and orange zest. Using a rubber scraper, spread the fruit butter mixture over the oatmeal mixture. Sprinkle with the remaining oatmeal mixture.

6. Bake for 30–35 minutes, or until the top is golden brown. Transfer the dish to a cooling rack and let cool completely before cutting into squares.

Exchanges / Choices
1 Carbohydrate

Calories	60	**Sodium**	20 mg
Calories from Fat	20	**Potassium**	40 mg
Total Fat	**2 g**	**Total Carbohydrate**	**10 g**
Saturated Fat	0 g	Dietary Fiber	1 g
Trans Fat	0 g	Sugars	4 g
Polyunsaturated Fat	0.5 g	**Protein**	**1 g**
Monounsaturated Fat	1 g	**Phosphorus**	**30 mg**
Cholesterol	**0 mg**		

CRANBERRY-PECAN BAKED PEACHES

Serves 4 / Serving Size: 2 peach halves and 2 tablespoons cranberry mixture

Fresh peaches are halved and baked with a tantalizing blend of dried cranberries and finely chopped pecans. Serve this dessert, with its roasted, concentrated flavors, for a round of applause at the end of your meal. *(See photo insert.)*

Cooking spray

1 1/2 tablespoons honey

1/3 cup sweetened dried cranberries

3 tablespoons finely chopped pecans

4 medium unpeeled peaches, nectarines, or pears, halved, pitted, and skin pierced in several places with a fork

2 teaspoons light tub margarine

1/2 teaspoon grated peeled gingerroot

Exchanges / Choices			
2 Fruit, 1 Fat			
Calories	**160**	**Sodium**	**15 mg**
Calories from Fat	45	**Potassium**	**320 mg**
Total Fat	**5 g**	**Total Carbohydrate**	**30 g**
Saturated Fat	0.5 g	Dietary Fiber	3 g
Trans Fat	0 g	Sugars	26 g
Polyunsaturated Fat	1.5 g	**Protein**	**2 g**
Monounsaturated Fat	2.5 g	**Phosphorus**	**45 mg**
Cholesterol	**0 mg**		

1. Preheat the oven to 350°F.

2. Lightly spray a 9-inch pie pan with cooking spray. Pour the honey into the pan. Heat the pan in the oven for 2 minutes, or until the honey is slightly runny. Remove from the oven, tilting the pan and swirling so the honey lightly coats the bottom.

3. Sprinkle the cranberries and pecans in the pan. Place the peaches with the cut side down over the cranberry mixture. (Some of the mixture may not be covered.) Cover the pan with aluminum foil. Bake for 30 minutes, or until the peaches are tender.

4. Arrange the peaches with the cut side up on a serving plate. Stir the margarine and gingerroot into the pan juices. Spoon the cranberry mixture into the cavities in the peaches. Spoon the pan juices over all. Serve warm or at room temperature.

FRESH FRUIT PARFAITS

Serves 4 / Serving Size: 1 cup fruit and 2 tablespoons sauce

This dessert takes on different personalities depending on the seasonal fruit you use. In the wintertime, try making the parfaits with apples, pears, and grapefruit and orange sections and using frozen unsweetened strawberries for the sauce.

Sauce

2 cups hulled strawberries (quartered if large)

2 tablespoons all-fruit seedless raspberry spread

1 tablespoon peach brandy or peach nectar

1/2 teaspoon almond extract

Fruit

1 cup blueberries

1 cup raspberries

1 cup sliced hulled strawberries

1 cup chopped peaches or nectarines

1. In a food processor or blender, process the sauce ingredients until smooth, stopping the motor once or twice to scrape down the sides of the bowl. Strain the sauce through a fine-mesh sieve for a smoother texture if desired.

2. Layer the fruit ingredients, in order, in parfait or wine glasses. Spoon the sauce over the fruits.

Exchanges / Choices
2 1/2 Fruit

Calories	140	**Sodium**	<5 mg
Calories from Fat	10	**Potassium**	310 mg
Total Fat	1 g	**Total Carbohydrate**	34 g
Saturated Fat	0 g	Dietary Fiber	6 g
Trans Fat	0 g	Sugars	24 g
Polyunsaturated Fat	0.5 g	**Protein**	1 g
Monounsaturated Fat	0 g	**Phosphorus**	45 mg
Cholesterol	**0 mg**		

TROPICAL LEMON GELATIN

Serves 6 / Serving Size: 1 wedge and 1/3 cup fruit

Traditional gelatin salad becomes new again when you add sweet summertime fruits and a creamy yogurt topping. Adding a bit of fresh lemon enhances the flavor of the gelatin and adds a tart freshness.

1 box (4-serving size) sugar-free lemon gelatin

1 cup boiling water

1/2 cup cold water

1 teaspoon grated lemon zest

1 tablespoon fresh lemon juice

1 cup fat-free vanilla yogurt

1 cup quartered hulled strawberries

1/2 cup diced mango

1 medium kiwifruit, peeled and sliced

1. Put the gelatin in a 9-inch glass pie pan or 8- or 9-inch square glass baking dish. Pour in the boiling water. Stir until the gelatin is completely dissolved.

2. Stir in the cold water and lemon juice. Cover with plastic wrap. Refrigerate until firm, at least 4 hours.

3. In a small bowl, stir the lemon zest into the yogurt. Spoon over the gelatin. Arrange the strawberries, mango, and kiwifruit decoratively on the yogurt mixture. Cut the gelatin into wedges or squares. Serve within 2 hours of adding the yogurt mixture for best results.

Cook's Tip on Zesting Citrus: It's easier to remove the zest of citrus fruits before squeezing out the juice. A rasp zester or grater works well. Just be careful and don't grate down to the bitter white layer of pith just below the peel.

Exchanges / Choices
1 Carbohydrate

Calories	70	Sodium	60 mg
Calories from Fat	10	Potassium	195 mg
Total Fat	**1 g**	**Total Carbohydrate**	**13 g**
Saturated Fat	0 g	Dietary Fiber	1 g
Trans Fat	0 g	Sugars	11 g
Polyunsaturated Fat	0 g	**Protein**	**3 g**
Monounsaturated Fat	0 g	**Phosphorus**	**90 mg**
Cholesterol	**<5 mg**		

MOCHA COOLER

Serves 4 / Serving Size: 3/4 cup

There's something about coffee that really enhances the already marvelous flavor of chocolate. You'll be convinced after only one sip of this cool, creamy drink that's also perked up with peppermint.

1 cup fat-free milk

2 cups frozen fat-free, sugar-free chocolate ice cream

2 tablespoons firmly packed dark brown sugar

1 tablespoon instant coffee granules

2 teaspoons vanilla extract

1/4 teaspoon peppermint extract

1–2 tablespoons coffee-flavored liqueur (optional)

Exchanges / Choices
2 Carbohydrate

Calories	160	**Sodium**	105 mg
Calories from Fat	0	**Potassium**	310 mg
Total Fat	0 g	**Total Carbohydrate**	30 g
Saturated Fat	0 g	Dietary Fiber	5 g
Trans Fat	0 g	Sugars	16 g
Polyunsaturated Fat	0 g	**Protein**	1 g
Monounsaturated Fat	0 g	**Phosphorus**	40 mg
Cholesterol	<5 mg		

1. In the order listed, put all the ingredients in a blender. Process until smooth. Serve immediately.

CREAMY FROZEN FRUIT WEDGES

Serves 8 / Serving Size: 1 wedge

This extremely easy, make-ahead dessert is perfect for the little kid in each of us. Simply toss a few ingredients together and pop the pie in the freezer. If you just can't wait, you can even eat it unfrozen. It will have a pudding-like consistency.

16 ounces frozen unsweetened sliced strawberries

1 1/2 cups fat-free vanilla yogurt

8 ounces crushed pineapple in its own juice, drained

2 cups frozen fat-free whipped topping, thawed in refrigerator

1. In a medium bowl, stir together the strawberries, yogurt, and pineapple.

2. Gently fold in the whipped topping. Spoon the mixture into a 9-inch pie pan. Cover with plastic wrap and freeze for 4 hours, or until the pie is firm.

3. About 15 minutes before serving, remove the pie from the freezer to let it thaw slightly before cutting into wedges.

Cook's Tip: When you need a really quick dessert, substitute fresh berries for the frozen ones. Combine the ingredients and skip the freezing step. Serve the strawberry mixture in chilled wine goblets.

Exchanges / Choices
1 Carbohydrate

Calories	80	Sodium	40 mg
Calories from Fat	10	Potassium	210 mg
Total Fat	**1 g**	**Total Carbohydrate**	**18 g**
Saturated Fat	0.5 g	Dietary Fiber	2 g
Trans Fat	0 g	Sugars	13 g
Polyunsaturated Fat	0 g	**Protein**	**3 g**
Monounsaturated Fat	0 g	**Phosphorus**	**70 mg**
Cholesterol	**<5 mg**		

MINTED FRUIT ICE

Serves 8 / Serving Size: 1/2 cup

This cold and refreshing dessert is bursting with fabulous fruit and a touch of aromatic fresh mint. The only difficulty is deciding whether to make it icy or to add the extra juice to make it creamy in texture.

1 cup 100% pineapple juice or fresh orange juice

1/4 cup sugar

2 teaspoons chopped fresh mint

1 teaspoon grated lime zest

2 tablespoons fresh lime juice

2 cups hulled strawberries, quartered if large

2 peaches or nectarines, peeled and coarsely chopped

1 medium banana

3 tablespoons 100% pineapple juice or fresh orange juice (optional)

1. In a small stainless steel saucepan, bring 1 cup pineapple juice, the sugar, mint, and lime zest to a boil over medium heat. Boil for 1 minute, stirring frequently. Pour into a medium bowl.

2. Fill a large bowl with ice cubes. Place the bowl with the pineapple juice mixture on the ice. Let the juice cool for 15–20 minutes, or until it comes to room temperature.

3. In a food processor or blender, process the remaining ingredients except the remaining 3 tablespoons pineapple juice until smooth, stopping the motor once or twice to scrape down the sides of the bowl. With the motor running, pour the pineapple juice mixture through the feed tube. Process until blended.

4. Pour into an 11 x 7 x 2-inch metal pan. Cover the pan with aluminum foil or plastic wrap and freeze for 2–3 hours, or until the edges of the fruit ice are hard.

5. Break it up in the pan and transfer it back to the food processor or blender. Process to the consistency of crushed ice. Or add the remaining pineapple juice and process for 2 minutes, or until creamy.

6. Serve immediately or transfer to an airtight freezer container and freeze. About 15–20 minutes before serving, remove from the freezer to thaw slightly.

Cook's Tip: Use a zester or rasp grater to remove the zest from citrus fruits. Zesters are tools that have small holes at one end. Pull the zester over the outer layer of the fruit to create thin strands of the colored rind.

Exchanges / Choices

1 1/2 Fruit

Calories	90	Sodium	<5 mg
Calories from Fat	5	Potassium	230 mg
Total Fat	0.5 g	Total Carbohydrate	21 g
Saturated Fat	0 g	Dietary Fiber	2 g
Trans Fat	0 g	Sugars	17 g
Polyunsaturated Fat	0 g	Protein	1 g
Monounsaturated Fat	0 g	Phosphorus	23 mg
Cholesterol	0 mg		

Index